We the People Are Failing

And must amend by popular vote the Declaration of Independence and our Constitution

&

Here is how

AS RESEARCHED
by
HEALTH SYSTEMS INSTITUTE INC.

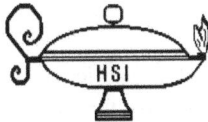

by

John R. Krismer, MHA-LFACHE

Principle Investigator

CCB Publishing
British Columbia, Canada

We the People Are Failing

Copyright ©2018, 2019 by John R. Krismer
ISBN-13 978-1-77143-355-6
First Edition, Revised

Library and Archives Canada Cataloguing in Publication
Krismer, John R., 1927-, author
We the People are failing / by John R. Krismer -- First edition.
Issued in print and electronic formats.
ISBN 978-1-77143-355-6 (softcover).--ISBN 978-1-77143-356-3 (pdf)
Additional cataloguing data available from Library and Archives Canada

Cover artwork credit: Deborah Barnett, Bozeman, Montana

Publisher: CCB Publishing
             British Columbia, Canada
             www.ccbpublishing.com

Dedicated to every American who wants to change the treacherous direction this Democracy has been forced to follow by an out of control and dysfunctional Congress and President, who are intentionally splitting this globalized Democracy into a Fascist controlled Banker's Cartel. And more recently, on October 7th, 2016, a complex Russian cyber-attack occurred that has led this once great nation into a *"Constitutional Crisis"* for the entire world of fearful Democratic Allies to watch.

Contents

Contents

Preface & An Important History

Following World War II, the U.S. Congress was nonpartisan, often providing bipartisan support in solving nonprofit issues that required multi-party cooperation. However, in the 1960s, political polarization began to increase as wealthy corporate financial donations influenced selected congressional members on profit issues involving health insurance and pharmaceutical products. These two issues presented a serious problem for Congress regarding healthcare policies and standards when both parties were trying to enact nonprofit Medicare and Medicaid versus the profit-seeking McCarran Ferguson Act — which forced this nation toward today's constitutional crisis. At that time the Duopoly Multi-party Congress also began to use partisanship tactics on issues they'd previously compromised on, such as the very successful single nonprofit Blue Cross Blue Shield noninsurance healthcare prepayment program they'd unanimously approved previously. However, once Congress became familiar with this new powerful corporate marketing tool that provided a source of additional congressional income for favors, they chose profit healthcare insurance, thereby becoming the only healthcare program in the world that sought profit from the sick and disabled. As a result, health care facilities had to make enormous budgetary adjustments at a time when they'd previously been successfully functioning as a nonprofit service without any need for profit spiraling healthcare costs out of control. In 1979, former President Gerald Ford reviewed this issue with this author, and we discussed how, as President, he was then forced to balance what he referred to as his "Iron Cross."

In World War II, the Nazi "Iron Cross" was used to identify strength, which prompted Congress to support a strong standard that every President would maintain a fair balance between all powers in the U.S., which became known as the President's "Iron Cross." The head of the "Iron Cross" represented the **People**, while the other three ends of the cross represented **Politicians**, the **Lobbyist Factions**, the **Bureaucracies**, and the **Armed Forces**, all of which the president was required to keep in balance. However, today's Congressional battles completely ignore the Iron Cross, and this hasn't been the first time this nation's conservative and liberal Duopoly Multi-party system has failed. Following the British War of 1812, this nation became involved in this same *"Partisan Extremism,"* which at that time caused the U.S. to eliminate the Duopoly problem by ushering in a "Single Congressional" body to represent the people. This single people party resulted in one of the longest successful political periods in this nation history, which became known as the *"Era of Good Feelings."* Then in the 1850s, a Duopoly Multi-party system was re-established for a second time between Andrew Jackson's "Democratic" party and Henry Clay's Republican "Whig" party. As a result, Congress is now substantially profiting from this nation's once tax-supported sick and disabled benefit, which has led to today's constitutional crisis. Because of this, Congress is also having far more difficulty passing bills or laws that improve one's equality as a U.S. citizen. And worse yet, with today's "Republican Party in Power, the Executive branch has suddenly chosen to no longer serve as a balancing factor, under what was originally designed to help bring all political parties together.

Then on top of all this, in the year 2000, this nation's Supreme Court, rather than the people, unwisely helped to destroy this political balancing act when the Court politically (not legally) appointed a Republican Presidential candidate. This new President, completely disregarded the important purpose of the "Iron Cross, resulting in today's bitter bipartisan battles. A good example of how this extreme "Illegal Partisanship" occurred is how the Republican Party now meets routinely in secret behind closed doors to plan and implement their *"Healthcare Act."* Thereby by ignoring this long-standing bipartisan rule of Congress, their Oath of Office, the Constitution, and this Iron Cross standard, they've also split the voting population — as well as eliminating any bilateral democratic participation.

The United States Democratic Party and the Republican Party have for a second time become completely dysfunctional, just as they previously did in the early eighteen hundreds. However, the Founding Fathers of the U.S. Constitution had anticipated this problem where a country could be taken over by corrupting forces, and therefore, the writers of the Constitution wanted the U.S. to be nonpartisan. **Federalist No. 10**, identified as *"Publius — the tenth"* of *"The Federalist Papers"* is a series of essays published on November 29, 1787, by James Madison — and later promoted by Alexander Hamilton who argued for their ratification in the U.S. Constitution. No. 10 was the most important of all American political writings in that it warned:

> *"... to guard against various factions of mankind, or groups of citizens whose interests are contrary to the rights of others or the interests of communities such as having differing opinions; differing amounts of wealth; or owning differing amounts of property." (1)*

On July 4, 1776, the thirteen United States of America's Congress unanimously approved the Declaration of Independence saying:

> *"— That to secure these rights, Governments are instituted among Men, deriving their just powers from the consent of the governed, — That whenever any Form of Government becomes destructive of these ends, it is the Right of the People to alter or to abolish it, and to institute new Government, laying its foundation on such principles and organizing its powers in such form, as to them shall seem most likely to effect (affect) their Safety and Happiness. Prudence, indeed, will dictate that Governments long established should not be changed for light and transient causes; and accordingly(,) all experience hath shewn (shown) that mankind are (is) more disposed to suffer, while evils are sufferable than to right themselves by abolishing the forms to which they are accustomed. But when a long train of abuses and usurpations, invariably pursuing the same Object evinces a design to reduce them under absolute Despotism, it is their right, it is their duty, to throw off such Government, and to provide new Guards for their future security." (2)*

As a result, the Declaration of Independence provides the people the right to gain control over such dysfunctional situations. It should, therefore, allow the people to conduct a popular vote when desired, to throw off such threatening issues. The people can also change the long-standing abuses of this Congress that have taken so many citizens "rights" away through nonpartisanship tactics. As a veteran, I'm embarrassed by the technologies that have replaced our ability to decide things for ourselves since this loss of the greatest generation that helped this country earn a ranking of first place in world leadership. Worse yet, we no longer can make a decision based on just *"common sense"* - like firing a President, or solving the following major crises that have urgently needed correction for a very long time:

For Example:

The U.S.'s financial panic of 1897 caused the creation of a privately held Commission to resolve the financial crisis that later confronted the U.S. Congress in the year 1907, while the United States still had no central bank. The creation of this privately held Commission resulted in a permanent ***"privately owned"*** Federal Reserve Banking Board being created to control the U.S. Treasury's financial resources. Worse yet, in 1921 the Congress allowed this independent Federal Reserve Banking Board to incorporate worldwide, becoming the very powerful *"Council of Foreign Relations (CFR),"* over which "We the People" have little or no financial control. Congressman Louis T. McFadden, Chairman of the U.S. House Banking and Currency Committee described this Crisis in 1934 in the 75th Congressional Record 1295-12603 when he stated:

> *"We have in this country one of the most corrupt institutions the world has ever known. I refer to the Federal Reserve Board and the Federal Reserve Banks. Some people think the Federal Reserve Banks are U.S. government institutions. They are not government institutions. They are private credit monopolies; domestic swindlers, rich and predatory money lenders which prey upon the people of the United States for the benefit of themselves and foreign customers. The Federal Reserve banks are the agents of the foreign central banks. The truth is the Federal Reserve Board has usurped the Government of the United States by the arrogant credit monopoly which operates the Federal Reserve Board."(3)*

In 1907, this Board included:

John Pierpont Morgan who was one of the most powerful bankers of that time, financed railroads and helped organize U.S. Steel, General Electric and other major corporations. Today, JPMorgan Chase & Co. is a multinational investment bank and financial service that is located in New York City and is the largest bank in the U.S. and one of the largest banks in the world.

John Davison Rockefeller Sr. was the founder of the Standard Oil Company, and the Rockefeller family is one of today's wealthiest philanthropic families. Rockefeller Sr. was an American oil industry magnate.

Paul Warburg was a partner in the banking firm of M.M. Warburg and Company in Hamburg, Germany in 1895, which was founded by his great-grandfather. In 1902, he moved to New York City to join his father-in-law's company as a partner overseeing international government loans. He recommended the establishment of the US central bank under a U.S. National Monetary Commission, established following the 1907 financial panic. Warburg was one of six men that created this country's plan for a National Reserve Association, which is so aptly described in the *"The Creature from Jekyll Island"* by Edward Griffin.

Otto Hermann Kahn was a banker and patron of the arts who played an important role in reorganizing the properties of six railroad systems, including the Union Pacific, and the Baltimore and Ohio U.S. railroad systems. Kahn worked in the London branch of Berlin's Deutsche Bank when the banking house of Speyer & Co. offered him a position in New York City, and by 1897 he became a partner in Kuhn, Loeb & Co. Many companies relied on Kahn's financial ability, and he successfully supported many Allied war efforts financially during World War I.

Jacob Henry Schiff was a banker, businessman, and philanthropist. He helped finance the expansion of American railroads and the Japanese military efforts in the Russo-Japanese War. He migrated to the U.S. following the Civil War and worked for the Kuhn, Loeb & Company on major Jewish issues involving American and international anti-Semitism, the care of needy Jewish immigrants, and the rise of Zionism. He also became a director of many important corporations, including the National City Bank of New York, Equitable Life Assurance Society, Wells Fargo & Company, and the Union Pacific Railroad.

The secret meeting on Jekyll Island:
In 1910, Senator Nelson Aldrich from Rhode Island, New Jersey was one of the most powerful Senators in Washington, D.C. and his son-in-law was John D, Rockefeller, Jr. Senator Aldrich served as the political spokesman for big business, while also serving as an investment associate for J.P, Morgan. Aldrich held extensive financial assets in banking,

manufacturing, and public utilities and he was the one that coordinated a secret meeting on Jekyll Island, off the coast of Georgia. Seven highly qualified and powerful financial advisors were assembled on Jekyll Island by the prospective members of this *"National Monetary Commission"* with the sole purpose of developing their secret plan for a privately held *"U.S. Federal Reserve."* This *"National Monetary Commission"* at that time represented one-fourth of the total wealth of the entire world and these representatives initially met at a New Jersey railroad station on a bitterly cold night in November 1910, traveling with Aldrich on his private railroad passenger car to Jekyll Island for a trumped-up nine-day duck hunting venture. However, instead of duck hunting, these seven men secretly drafted their plan for a privately held *U.S. Federal Reserve.* These seven men that were assigned to develop this authoritarian cartel's plan with Nelson Aldrich included:

- *Abraham Platt Andrew, Assistant Secretary of the U, S. Treasury;*
- *Frank A. Vanderlip, president of the National City Bank of New York, representing William Rockefeller and the international investment banking house of Kuhn, Loeb, and Company;*
- *Henry P. Davison, senior partner of the J.P. Morgan Company;*
- *Charles D. Norton, president of J.P. Morgan's First National Bank of New York:*
- *Benjamin Strong, Head of J.P. Morgan's Banker's Trust Company;*
- *Paul M. Warburg. Partner in Kuhn, Loeb & Company, a representative of the Rothschild banking dynasty in England and France, and brother of Max Warburg who was head of the Warburg banking consortium in Germany and the Netherlands. (4)*

What's most shocking about today's U.S. *Federal Reserve* is that it has now become nothing more than a *"Banker's Cartel"* that remains owned by these private international investors that are becoming very wealthy and are not subject to the U.S. citizen's oversight.

Note: A cartel is a group of independent businesses that join together to coordinate the production, pricing, or marketing of their customers. The purpose of a cartel is to reduce competition and thereby increase profitability through a shared monopoly, forcing the industry to pay higher prices than through free competition or enterprise.

"We the People" may never be able to regain control over this treacherous autocratic group that this once successful Democracy is now being forced to follow. And yet "We the People" created this democracy for citizens that sought fairness instead of European Cartel types of control, extreme wealth or property ownership, suppression, dictatorships, fascism or authoritarianism from which the U.S. citizens are now seeking to escape. "We the People" were seeking freedom; equality; ethics; morality and honesty for all citizens that pledged allegiance to the United States of America, and yet today there are no more places that "We the People" can escape too. What "We the People" want is a democratically elected government in which the supreme power was vested in the people. A power that can be exercised by the people involving both a profit system that is fairly taxed and a non-profit tax-supported system that provides education, healthcare, infrastructure, and protective societal benefits at the lowest possible price - thereby assuring political equality in place of a socialistic controlled government.

In 1932, a total overthrow of the United States Democracy by this Cartel attempted to unseat President Franklin Delano Roosevelt (FDR) before his first term in office. However, this Cartel's take over was publicly exposed by retired Marine Corps Major General Smedley Butler, at the 1934 McCormack-Dickstein Congressional Committee meeting. In Butler's testimony he told the committee that on July 17, 1932, he was approached by several wealthy members of this cartel to help *"overthrow this nation's democracy"* by a military coup. In the Congressional Committee's report, it validated Butler's allegations, but no prosecutions or further investigations ever followed, which is what usually happens when it involves any member of this exclusive upper crust. At that time, however, the devastation of the Great Depression was causing many of these very rich cartel families to question the foundation of our Democracy, considering Fascism, Socialism, Dictatorships or Communism as an alternative that would give them greater control over their wealth — rather than a Democracy that protects everyone's equality. By 1935, most of the Republicans, bankers and large corporations also openly opposed FDR's "New Deal." As a result, FDR was forced to abandon the gold standard because of the Great Depression, and this became an ideal time for this privately owned banking system to acquire the potential of earning unlimited interest from the valueless paper money they were able to create with a stroke of the pen. Worse yet, without a gold standard, there was no way to protect one's savings should inflation occur. Other countries were also forced to float their unregulated currencies since this nation's global currency was no longer backed by U.S. gold. Gold had previously served as one's protector of property rights, but now this uncontrolled deficit spending allowed this banker's scheme to acquire and control the global wealth just as the CFR had planned. On the positive side, however, this attempt at a Smedley's coup did unknowingly expose the CFR's secret long-range *"Grand Design Plan"* for their eventual financial rule over the entire world. More importantly, the paper money the Federal Reserve created at will was earning this Cartel huge interest profits. Because of this, the international banks next needed to find someone to take the fall when any loaner failed to pay their loan. To acquire such a fall guy, the CFR shrewdly negotiated an agreement with the U.S. Treasury to authorize the Congressional approval of Federal Grants, to protect the Cartel's privately owned banks from going bankrupt and thereby destroying their new world economy. Few people realized or cared that the U.S. citizen's who unknowingly paid this nation's taxes became the fall guy for these privately owned banks.

Worse yet, by ignoring presidential credentials or job description criteria, as well as one's personal and financial qualifications, the Congress is now blindly sanctioning far too many unqualified candidates to run for President of the United States. Two of the last three elections have placed two unqualified Presidents in this office through the "Electoral College" rather than by the people's "Popular Vote" for one of the most important offices in the world.

President Lincoln wrote in his Gettysburg Address on Nov. 19, 1863:

> *"Four score and seven years ago, our fathers brought forth on this continent, a new nation, conceived in Liberty, and dedicated to the proposition that all men are created equal ... that this nation, under God, shall have a new birth of freedom — and that government of the people, by the people, for the people, shall not perish from the earth."(2)*

In 1887, Professor Joseph Olson, often misrepresented as Alexander Tyler, a Scottish history professor at the University of Edinburgh, said regarding the fall of the Athenian Republic:

> *"Democracy is always temporary; it simply cannot exist as a permanent form of government. A democracy will continue to exist up until the time that voters discover that they can vote themselves generous gifts from the public treasury. From that moment on, the majority always votes for the candidates who promise the most benefits from the public treasury, with the result that every democracy will finally collapse over loose fiscal policy, (which is) always followed by a dictatorship. The average age of the world's greatest civilizations from the beginning of history has been about 200 years. During those 200 years, these nations always progressed through the following sequence:*
>
> > *From bondage to spiritual faith;*
> > *From spiritual faith to great courage;*
> > *From courage to liberty;*
> > *From liberty to abundance;*
> > *From abundance to complacency;*
> > *From complacency to apathy;*
> > *From apathy to dependence;*
> > *From dependence, back into bondage."(3)*

Just as wealth destroyed the first Democracy in Athens, it has once again become the number one obstacle to the U.S. remaining a Democracy, which protects the equality of *"We the People."* This book provides facts and speaks openly on the many areas this unsupervised Congress has failed regarding their "Oath of Office" under the current ridiculous Duopoly system that has for the second time brought this nation to its knees. The U.S. urgently needs to face up to the fact that the wealthy one percent is now posing the greatest threat the U.S. has ever experienced. There have been many major Congressional mistakes made during the twentieth century that could end the greatest democracy this world has ever known if "We the People" of the United States are not allowed a vote to make these major changes recommended in Chapter One by a popular vote of the people. Only then will there be a thread of a chance that "We the People" can salvage our Democracy. However, if the people's popular vote allows this *"Illegal Partisan Extremism"* to continue, this Democracy will be doomed to failure. Even then, to even have a slight chance of success, the major Amendments outlined in "Section

One" must be voted on by the citizens of the United States by popular vote so "We the People" can then enforce the many necessary changes required. Only after accomplishing this, will the people of this great nation even have a chance to evaluate and take action once again at their state level. Only then will they have a chance to implement their decisions regarding the many facts outlined in the remaining chapters of this book — thereby reinstating the necessary changes for the ongoing democratic leadership that the rest of the world can once again trust.

1 *Federalist Papers No. 10*, identified as *"Publius — the tenth"* of *"The Federalist Papers,"* is a series of essays that was published on November 29, 1787, by James Madison

2 The United States Constitution

3 McFadden, Louis T. *The Federal Reserve Corporation, remarks in Congress.* Boston: Forum Publication Co. 1934.

4 Bagwell, Tyler E. *Images of America: The Jekyll Island Club.* Charleston, SC: Arcadia, 1998), 18-19 pp

SECTION I
RECOMMENDED POPULAR VOTE AMENDMENTS

We need to appropriately Amend the Declaration of Independence or Constitution as required by popular vote to recover our Democracy. Here is how.

1

Recommended Popular Vote

PROPOSED AMENDMENT ONE:
The issuance of Executive Order 11110 on June 4, 1963, was an effort by President J.F. Kennedy to take back this nation's power from the Federal Reserve and transfer it back to the United States Department of the Treasury. James Marr's book *"Crossfire"* confirmed this order. However, the current Multi-party Congress, coupled with this private global commission, is now causing a *"Global Constitutional Crisis"* for this country's once *"Greatest Democracy in the world."*

Executive Order 11110 by President John F. Kennedy stated:

"By the authority vested in me by section 301 of title 3 of the United States Code, it is ordered as follows:

SECTION 1. Executive Order No. 10289 of September 19, 1951, as amended, is hereby further amended –

(a) By adding at the end of paragraph 1 thereof the following subparagraph (j):
(j) The authority vested in the President by paragraph (b) of section 43 of the Act of May 12, 1933, as amended (31 U.S.C. 821 (b)), to issue silver certificates against any silver bullion, silver, or standard silver dollars in the Treasury not then held for redemption of any outstanding silver certificates, to prescribe the denominations of such silver certificates, and to coin standard silver dollars and subsidiary silver currency for their redemption," and
(b) By revoking subparagraphs (b) and (c) of paragraph 2 thereof.

SECTION 2. The amendment made by this Order shall not affect any act done, or any right accruing or accrued, or any suit or proceeding had or commenced in any civil or criminal cause before the date of this Order but all such liabilities shall continue and may be enforced as if said amendments had not been made.

Signed by:
John F Kennedy, White House" (1)

Executive Order 11110 was the first and only proposed Amendment to take this nation's financial authority back and strip the Federal Reserve Bank of its power to loan valueless money that was created by the stroke of a pen at an extremely high rate of interest to the U.S. government. What's so surprising about Executive Order 11110 is it has never been repealed and is still *"legally valid."*

Shockingly, President John F. Kennedy was assassinated five months after his Executive Order was approved, and worse yet, as of January 1, 2019, this Kennedy effort has been the only real attempt ever made to return the power to issue real-valued currency by the U.S. government. This country's current spiraling debt of $21.97 trillion, as of December 31, 2018, is largely due to the high-interest rate Americans currently pay the Federal Reserve through our current tax dollars. President Kennedy's order also gave the U.S. Treasury the power to issue silver certificates against any silver, silver bullion, or standard silver dollars in the Treasury. For every ounce of silver in the U.S. Treasury, Kennedy's order also restricted the government from placing any more valueless money into circulation, and his order successfully placed nearly $4.3 billion in U.S. silver backed notes into circulation. The ramifications of this Bill were enormous, for with the stroke of the cartel's pen, they were able to place valueless paper money into circulation. And President Kennedy was on his way to putting the Federal Reserve Bank of New York out of business if enough of these silver certificates had been allowed to come into circulation and that would have eliminated the current demand for high-interest Federal Reserve notes. Why? Because the silver certificates were to be backed by silver and the Federal Reserve Cartel's notes had no value or backing of any kind. Yes, Executive Order 11110 could have prevented the U.S. national debt from reaching its current out of control level. It also would have given the government the ability to repay its debt without

4

going to the Federal Reserve and being charged interest in creating this Cartel's valueless money. However, for some unknown reason, after Mr. Kennedy's assassination, the Treasury issued no more silver certificates.

Interestingly, this Executive Order has never been used by any other U.S. President even though this Kennedy Bill is still valid. Almost all of this U.S. taxpayer debt has occurred since 1963, and if the U.S. had continued this Executive Order 11110, this national debt would be nowhere near its current level. President Kennedy had challenged the most successful intermediary that has ever been used to drive up world debt and support so many costly wars financially. Kennedy's Executive Order 11110 would have severely cut into the huge profits and control of this powerful New York Banking Cartel that currently controls and finances a majority of all loans and supports most wars throughout the entire world.

An Amendment to activate this Executive Order 11110 regarding the return of the fiscal responsibility to the U.S. Treasury is of vital importance to our Democracy.

PROPOSED AMENDMENT TWO:

Another major area where we as a nation can no longer make a decision based on just **common sense** is the **Dysfunctional Duopoly Multi-Party Congress** that has now failed this nation for a second time. History has determined that wealthy factions and wars are the most common cause of all democracies failing within 200 years. The first U.S. failure occurred after the 1812 war with the British when that era saw the collapse of the first U.S. Duopoly Multi-party Democratic-Republican system. And now, today, these same selfish, bitter partisan disputes between these same two Congressional parties have for a second time brought the U.S. to its knees. In reviewing the world history, the first democracy of ancient Athens, Greece was a *"**Nonpartisan Direct Democracy.**" In a Direct Democracy,* all the eligible citizens vote on laws rather than electing someone to do this for them. The *"Founding Fathers"* of our U.S. Constitution also wanted the U.S. government to be nonpartisan. However, as previously described by James Madison in *Federalist, No. 10,* the most important of all American political writings, predicted humanity would inherently form informal alliances with those who sought differing opinions; differing amounts of wealth or owned differing amounts of property that worked against the public's interests - thereby disregarded the universal rights of citizens.

In *Federalist No. 9*, Alexander Hamilton said:

> *"...a firm Union will be of the utmost moment to the peace and liberty of the States as a barrier against domestic faction and insurrection."(2)*

Although the "Founding Fathers" did not expect the U.S. ever to become partisan, James Madison understood that these types of informal organizations could become a threat, so he recommended incorporating both *"Conservative" and "Liberal"* principles into **"one"** at both the **national** and **state** level to represent the local citizens better. No. 10 had also recommended that the heads of state (Presidents) should remain neutral regarding partisan politics. However, the U.S. has now allowed another Duopoly Multi-party system, which disregards Madison's single people party system. Not too long ago the Congress also established an *"Iron Cross policy,"* which required every President keep the **Politicians**, the **Lobbyist Factions**, the **Bureaucracies**, and the **Armed Forces** in balance. But this *"Iron Cross policy"* has now been intentionally disregarded by today's Republican President. The Duopoly Multi-party politics had failed for the first time from 1816 to 1829, forcing the people to reorganize into a single successfully identified people-oriented party which became known as the *"Era of Good Feelings."* However, by 1850, partisan politics had once again resurfaced between Andrew Jackson's "Democratic" party and Henry Clay's Republican "Whig" party. Ironically, this same type of Duopoly Multi-party system has for a second time split the two parties. This time the split has reached a point where the Democratic and Republican parties refuse to even meet in the same room. Under today's two-party system, the parties do not even want to discuss any other options than their "Liberal" or "Conservative" issues depending on which party is in the majority. It is this split into either liberal or conservative issues rather than the people issues that have caused today's two-party system to become so dysfunctional.

Wealthy factions have long felt they could best protect their wealth under a *"Fascist Dictatorship"* where they do not have to treat the people equally. Under this Multi-party type of system, one of the parties holds the majority in the legislature and is referred to as the *"Majority Party"* while the other party becomes the *"Minority Party."* This Majority/Minority type of system has now become a huge problem during the last three presidential elections. During those three terms, the conservative and liberal parties reached a point where neither party would concede any policy change to the other party, which of course puts an end to any form of *bilateral diplomacy* that can benefit the people as a whole. In fact, each party ping-ponged the other party's liberal or conservative policies when they were in power, ignoring their *"Oath of Office"* that each member of Congress took to represent the people under the U.S. Constitution which states:

> *"I do solemnly swear (or affirm) that I will support and defend the Constitution of the United States against all enemies foreign and domestic; that I will bear true faith and allegiance to the same; that I take this obligation freely, without any mental reservation or purpose of evasion; and that I will well and faithfully discharge the duties of the office on which I am about to enter: So help me God."*

And now the super-wealthy one percent of the U.S. population is regularly providing financial kickbacks (inducements or bribes) to this failed two-party system. It is these money bribes that are the root cause of what has brought this country to a halt, and which now urgently demands that *"We the People"* regain supervisory control of all political salaries and benefits at the state level. Isn't it ironic that the U.S. Senate and House of Representatives are all appointed by the people at the state level and then moved to the national level with almost no control or supervision? Therefore this loss of supervision over the House and Senate's complex Duopoly Multi-party system has inherently become the number one problem for the people of this country, which suggests each state must urgently regain control over the Senate and the House's payroll if this nation ever intends to recover its democracy.

In January 2016 Michael Coblenz published an article in *"The Hill"* when the U.S. was facing numerous problems that dealt with racial discrimination, terrorism, and their inability to even approve the government's budget, which prompted him to say:

> *"The two-party system is destroying America. Democrats and Republicans are in a death match, and the American people are caught in the middle."(3)*

Michael J. Dowd also published an article in the Wall Street Journal indicating that the evolution of the 2016 election has shown that the two major parties are going to have to deal with this multi two-party system both locally and at the state level.

This nation's *"first single-party people system,"* the *"Era of Good Feeling,"* was created to unify all Americans. However, today's Congress is once again right back where the U.S. was in 1829 — where the politicians have become the number one obstacle to the U.S. remaining a Democracy that protects the equality of "We the People." Worse yet, this democracy will perish from the earth if this nation is unable to resist what's currently happening to what was once the greatest Democracy in the world. History has shown that very wealthy people best exist under a *"Fascist Dictatorship"* where a nation does not profess to treat people equally. Wealthy plutocratic and corporate control most often attacks democracies at the national or international level — while people power in a democracy can be best accomplished at the local community or state level. Isn't it ironic that the U.S. Senate and House of Representatives are all appointed by the people at the state level and then moved to the national level with almost no control? Because the state that appoints them does not pay this unsupervised Congress, the Congressional members are entirely free to manage and improperly administer the federal tax dollars they pay to themselves. Such unbridled employee freedom defies all employer/ employee standards, and because of this, the people have lost control over both the House and Senate. On top of all this, the citizens of the U.S. have never really approved the powerful (CFR) that still privately owns this country's Federal Reserve; the wealthy corporate plutocrats and their skilled lobbyists; the "Citizens United" and the more recently created "Super PACS" that provide financial benefits to selected congressional members for favors. Therefore this loss of control by the people over the House and Senate's complex Duopoly Multi-party system has inherently become a number one problem for the people of this country and is once again destroying America. Democrats and Republicans are in a death match, with the American people caught in the middle. A 2015 Gallop Polls suggested the people were seriously seeking a change in political parties. Maybe it took 247 years for the U.S. to find out that democracies need the people at the state's level to manage the politicians they appoint to represent them in the House and the Senate — just as they previously did when the people amended the Constitution to create the "Era of Good Feelings," from 1816 until 1850.

PROPOSED AMENDMENT THREE:

A third major area that added to the U.S's destruction of our democracy involved the **Globalization of both Democracies and Dictatorships as one** without **written Policy or Procedures.** When George H. W. Bush Sr. was appointment as CIA Director, this was probably when the *Shrub Dynasty* first took root. Then later, as Vice President under President Reagan, and then as President of the United States for one term, H.W. became the *"Overlord" of the "Shrub Dynasty,"* and that was when he openly introduced to the public the term *"New World Order"* in his State of the Union Address, on January 31, 2002, when he said:

> *"What is at stake is more than one small country, it is a big idea - a new World order to achieve the universal aspirations of humankind based on shared principles and the rule of law. The winds of change are with us now."(4)*

Establishing a *"New World Order"* was a very premature undertaking in that the U.S. had only recently become a world leader in Democracy. The U.S. was not about to become a small nation in a multi-political world that would inherently unite and become one happy family of people, entrepreneurs, religions, and ethnic groups while ignoring each country's inherent political control and pride. In any event, the wealthy Fascistic controlled governments were far too anxious to expand their corporate marketing before they had approved proper written policy and procedures that Bush referred to as *"shared principles and the rules of law."* Implementing *"shared principles and the rules of law"* has now proven next to impossible in today's *"Constitutional Crisis,"* which both the world and the U.S. are experiencing. However, Bush's new *"World Order"* did unknowingly exposed the CFR's plan to replace this country's democracy with their *"Grand Design"* for their nondemocratic rule over the entire world. The CFR was far too anxious to expand their corporate marketing well before their controlled and poorly developed organizations like the United Nations (UN) and the North Atlantic Treaty Organization (NATO) had even the slightest chance to develop any *"shared principles or rules of law"* to protect *"We the People."* And as a result, the many costly *"Off Shore Tax Havens,"* and the increasing number of rampant corporate tax evasion programs now in danger every country in the world. In addition to all this, today's wealthy factions now financially control the U.S. Congress, which has become subservient to these powerful plutocratic factions and their skilled corporate lobbyists. As a result — today's congressional members now ignore the voices of the citizens of this once Great Democracy. By prematurely opening this door to these huge corporate markets, *"Globalization"* has been all about money, and now these highly competitive entrepreneurs will never willingly let any *"principles or rules of law"* reduce the huge profits they are currently earning. Worse yet, the U.S. Congress has become subservient to these plutocratic factions and their powerful corporate lobbyists. But the hard fact is *"We the People"* can no longer afford to pay for this fallacious and illegal type of *"Globalization,"* and "We the People" need to once again successfully reclaim this nation's independence by reasserting and reclaiming the freedom this nation once held sacred.

SUMMARY
This free democracy may well perish from the earth if *"We the People"* do not strongly resist what's currently happening to what was once the greatest Democracy in the world. This rapidly growing *"Enemy Within"* has now become the greatest enemy this democracy has ever faced. This political faction of *"Plutocrats"* that are buying off this nation's politicians and splitting this nation's population must be brought to an end if this nation is to accomplish people "equality" under a democracy.

It's now up to the people to demand these dysfunctional organizational crises that include the Federal Reserve Cartel; the Duopoly Multi-party Congress; the lack of Democratic Globalization Policies be amended by a popular vote of the citizens before the United States 2020 election. Only then can this wealthy faction of *"Plutocrats,"* as outlined in the Federalist Papers No. 10, that are buying off our politicians and intentionally splitting our nation come to an end. Only then, can "We the People" once again manage at the state level the policies involving the environment, education, healthcare, immigration, gun violence and the many other issues the people have to live with and that are described more factually in

Section II of this book.

This Author pitched baseball, and his catcher seldom called for a drop ball because the fastball would usually cause the batter to ground out or pop-up to the outfield, and the fastball was a most reliable pitch. However, he could also pitch an unbelievable drop ball that when thrown toward the batters head, it would end up in the catcher's mitt on the ground just behind home plate after it crossed the plate in the strike zone. He had been blessed with this amazing drop pitch because he'd broke his arm at 14 years of age and his arm was crooked at the elbow, allowing for this huge drop ball whenever he threw it. The pitch was virtually un-hittable, and his long-time catcher hated to call it because it was also very difficult to catch — so as a result, he seldom signaled for it since he could usually get through the entire game using variations of the fastball. One day, in a Championship game where the Author's team was leading 2 to 1 in the ninth inning — and with the head of the opponent's batter's order coming up to bat — this catcher called nine straight drop balls, and after nine strikes in a row, the Author's team won the game. However, the catcher only used this pitch in a very desperate situation.

Ironically this is kind of like the 247 years we've successfully lived under a people controlled democracy, where the U.S. has at times resolved world wars, depressions, and a variety of other unbelievable conflicts and problems. But now, more recently, every U.S. citizen is becoming very concerned that the people of this great nation have only one chance left to salvage the *"Greatest Democracy that ever existed"* by defeating this *"Autocratic Worldwide Grand Design Plan"* that is currently well on its way to taking over the entire world.

So isn't it time for *"We the People"* to throw that drop ball?

1 Executive Order 1111010289 by U.S. President John F. Kennedy on June 4, 1963

2 *Federalist Papers: No. 9:* The Union as a Safeguard Against Domestic Faction and Insurrection For the Independent Journal. Hamilton

3 http:// the hill.com/blogs/.../politics/267222-the-two-party-system-is-destroying-america jan 28,2016

4 *The State of the Union speech* January 31, 2002.: "Bush declares war on the world." www.bushwatch.com/archives-jan06.htm - 225k - Cached

SECTION II
FACTS ABOUT
OUR DEMOCRACY

2

House and Senate

Organization, Salaries, Benefits, and Donations:

The House of Representatives is referred to as the *"Lower House"* while the Senate is called the *"Upper House,"* forming two (bicameral) separate lawmaking assemblies that currently make up the legislature. The Members of the House of Representatives serve two-year terms, and many of the members are considered for reelection every even year, while the six Resident Commissioners from Washington D.C., American Samoa, Guam, Northern Mariana Islands, the U.S. Virgin Islands and Puerto Rico are non-voting members. These Resident Commissioners are not allowed to vote on proposed legislation in the full House but can participate in certain other House functions like voting in a committee of which they are a member, and where they can introduce legislation at those committee meetings. The Resident Commissioner of Puerto Rico is elected every four years while the other non-voting delegates are elected every two years. Senators serve six-year terms and elections to the Senate are staggered over seven years so that only about 1/3 of the Senate is up for reelection during an election year. The Senate serves six-year terms as a check on the House. The number of the House of Representatives (the lower Chamber) is based on each state's population and is responsible for representing the people of their state. The total number of voting members in the House is 435 by law. The House is composed of one member who represents each state's congressional district, which is allocated in each of the 50 states by the population as measured by the U.S. Census. Since the inception of the House of Representatives in 1789, all representatives were previously elected popularly while the presiding officer, the *"Speaker of the House,"* is elected by the members and traditionally serves as the leader of the majority party. The floor leaders are chosen by the Democratic Caucus or the Republican Conferences depending on who has the controlling number of votes. The House is hierarchically organized, with leadership roles such as the Majority Leader playing a larger part than the Minority leader. The rules and procedures used in the House of Representatives depend on a variety of customs, precedents, and traditions — and in many cases, the House waives some of its stricter rules including time limits on debates by unanimous consent. The U.S. House of Representative's composition and powers of the House are in Article One of the United States Constitution, and their duties include:

- *The House passes federal legislation such as having certain exclusive powers to initiate all bills related to revenue and spending bills, which, after concurrence by the Senate, are sent to the President for consideration.*
- *The power to collect tax money and other revenue*
- *The sole authority to impeach federal officials, and send them to the Senate for trial*
- *The authority to choose the President in an Electoral College deadlock*
- *The Constitution permits the House to expel a member with a two-thirds vote*
- *The House also has the power to censure or reprimand its members formally; censure or reprimanding a member requires only a simple majority and does not remove that member from office*

The United States Senate is the Upper Chamber of the U.S. Congress, and together with the House, they represent the Legislature of the United States. The Senate appoints two Senators for every state for a total of 100 members, which provides all 50 states equal representation by having approximately the same size of constituencies, other than some seven Senators that do have larger constituencies and therefore receive greater stature and recognition in the Senate. With longer terms and fewer members than the House, the Senate has traditionally been considered a less partisan chamber because it has fewer members than the House. The composition and powers of the Senate are in Article One of the United States Constitution, and their duties include:

- *The sole power of "advice and consent" in representing the states. These include the ratification of treaties, the confirmation of cabinet secretaries,*

Supreme Court Justices, Federal Judges and other federal executive officials, flag officers, regulatory officials, ambassadors, and other federal uniformed officers

- *In cases where no candidate receives a majority of elector votes for Vice-President, the Senate elects one of the top two recipients of electors for that office*

- *The responsibility of conducting trials of those impeached by the House.*

- *The Senate serves as a check on the regional, popular, and rapidly changing politics of the House,*

According to the *"Center for Responsive Politics (CRP),"* it has been noted that the median personal wealth for a member of Congress has grown from $785,515 in 2008 to $1.1 million in 2014. The net worth of a Senator has increased from $2.3 million to $2.8 million from 2007 to 2013, while the net worth of a member of the House increased from $708,500 to $843,507. For a family in the U.S. in 2013, this is significantly different than their median wealth of $56,356. Comparatively, this average annual income of a family in the U.S. has decreased from $58,003 in 2007 to $55,775 in 2015.

The Executive Director, of the *"International Agency,"* Winnie Byanyima, warned that this explosion in inequality is holding back the fight against global poverty at a time when 1 in 9 people do not have enough to eat and more than a billion people still live on less than $1.25 / day.

The *"International Policy Statement (IPS),"* reveals that the 400 richest Americans now have more wealth than the bottom 61 percent of the U.S. population.

The *"Forbes 400,"* reveals that just twenty individuals at the top, now control more wealth than the bottom half of the population and that's 152 million people living in 57 million households.

The debt of the United States, which is held by the people, was $13.62 trillion in 2018, or about 75% of the previous 12 months of GDP. Intra-governmental holdings stood at $5.34 trillion, giving a combined total gross national debt of $18.96 trillion in 2018. This mounting level of the U.S. government debt lacks the Congresses' incentive to solve. Many of this government's substantial pay increases in Congress have occurred during this country's economic downturn, which suggests that the politicians are not minding the store, but are more concerned with their salaries, donations, and benefits. Although the *"U.S. Office of Personnel Management"* prepares the Congresses' paychecks and finances their benefits program using federal tax dollars — the U.S. House of Representatives and the Senate completely manage their salary and benefit programs. Recently the CRP identified some 261 millionaire members in the United States' House of Representatives and the Senate. Worse yet, this nation's elected representatives are spending far too much time managing their re-election and their salary and benefit programs — instead of doing the full-time work they were hired to do by their state. Congressional Members completely politicize themselves as either a Liberal Democrat or a Conservative Republican and have become so dysfunctional that they can no longer even discuss or make decisions or appointments because the party in power at any given time opposes either a liberal or conservative decision. The fact is, the United States can no longer live with either a total conservative or liberal agenda. Political decisions have to deal with both conservative and liberal problems. Over the last eight years, Congress has ignored making any decisions because of this ridiculous split between the two parties that once made bipartisan decisions that were best for the people and not one party.

The cost allowance for the Congresses' double office system and a double staff costs **$723,964,675.00** annually in 2018 while averaging **$1,353,205.00** for each member.

The overall annual compensation programs for the United States' House of Representatives and the Senate are:

2018	Per-Member	Senate Total Annual
Hair Care	$333.87	$33,387.00
Restaurant Fund	$723.70	$72,370.12
Health and Fitness	$1,238.56	$123,856.74
Meal Cost	$2,766.99	$276,629.00
Photography-Studio	$659.15	$65,915.24
Recording Studio	$227.22	$22,722.52
Stationary Fund	$2988,21	$298,821.41
Total	$10,614.43	$1,060,385.29

- *Basic House and Senate salary – $174,000*
- *Majority and Minority Leaders in the House and Senate and the Chief Administrative Officer – $193,400*
- *President Pro Tempore and Speaker of the House– $223,500*
- *Vice President (President of the Senate) – $230,700*

The Budget for the House and Senate members in 2018 includes the base salary for each non-executive member of **$174,000.00** annually and the average annual individual expenses per Congressional member of **$256,574.00**. The following annual *"Personal Expenses"* per Senator per year were reported by: http://www.fms.treas.gov/annualre/index.html#agency

Senate -Personal Expenses - 2010

<u>The Cost-of-Living-Adjustment (COLA):</u>

- *COLA's automatically take effect annually if not repealed by Congress.*

Total expenses for the 535 House of Representatives and the Senate members for 2010 were estimated to be **$5,673,431.45** for each member – while costing the U.S. **$3,935,285,875.75** annually for the entire Congress, and this excludes the huge outside benefits Congress receives from various power factions outside of Congress.

Congressional members that filed their financial disclosure forms in 2013 indicated they cost the U.S. **$4.3 billion** annually, which would be equivalent to some 76,000 American households. And this ignores the COLA and their Civil Service perks; their Government Health Insurance for members and their family; their Retirement Benefits; and their Life Insurance. If the Congresses' financial disclosures are accurate, the Congress has informally increased their annual income totally out of reach, and this needs to be cut substantially and then supervised in the future.

The Civil Service Retirement Service (CSRS):

The CSRS was not designed to coordinate with Social Security, so in 1986 Congress created the *"Federal Employees' Retirement System Act (FERS)"* for all new members of Congress and Federal Employees. All the United States' House of Representatives and Senate Members elected since 1984 received FERS and those elected before 1984 CSRS. However, more recently, all members have been given the option of remaining with CSRS or switching to FERS. All Members of Congress fund their retirement through a combination of federal tax dollars and their contributions and that their retirement becomes fully vested after five years of participation. Today, Members of Congress under FERS contribute 1.3 percent of their salary into their retirement plan, and they do pay 6.2 percent of their salary to Social Security Tax, in which they chose *"not"* to participate. Perhaps one can now better understand why so many politicians are so very anxious to privatize Social Security. After completing 20 years of service, the members become eligible for a pension after they reach the age of 50, or at any age if they've completed 25 years of service or have reached the age of 62. All Members must have served five years to be eligible for a pension, and the amount of pension depends on their years of service based on the average of the highest three years of salary. However, the starting amount of a Member's Retirement Annuity may not exceed 80% of their final salary. Of those that have retired under CSRS – 344 are receiving an average annual pension of $74,136 while the 276 that retired under FERS –are receiving an average annual pension of $41,316 in 2018.

Health Insurance:

Health Insurance for the United States' House of Representatives and the Senate allows for a comprehensive *"Federal Employees Health Benefits program (FEHB)"* that allows each member to select from among several health benefit plans. It's important to note that this program is a government program that will not be transferred to some profit insurance corporation as many politicians are suggesting for Medicare and Medicaid, which they refer to as *"Socialistic."* Participation in their FHEB program is on a voluntary contributory basis and based on the program they select, they pay the lowest rates of any other health care program in the nation. Perhaps a single, cost-effective non-profit prepayment program could be considered for this nation's future *"Universal Healthcare System,"* or perhaps the Members of the United States' House of Representatives and Senate should receive what every citizen receives.

Life Insurance:

Life insurance for the United States' House of Representatives and Senate members are all eligible to participate in a very cost-effective *"Federal Employees Group Life Insurance Program."* The amount of coverage for personal insurance depends on the coverage they select. Here again, this outstanding program could be made available to every citizen of the U.S.

Allowances for Members' Representational Allowance (MRA):

The MRA is calculated based on Personnel, Official Office Expenses, and Official (Franked) Mail. The average House allowance ranges from $1,299 million to $1,638 million per member, while the Senate ranges from $2,758 million to $4,417 million. These allowances vary based on the size of the member's state.

Outside Earned Income Limits and Prohibition on Honoraria:

All outside income for the United State's House of Representatives and Senate was recently reduced by the Ethics Reform Committee, limiting honoraria to 27% of salary. The permissible "outside earned income" is limited to 15% of the base annual pay level of the Executive Salary Schedule. Certain types of outside earned income are prohibited:

- *Congressional members may not receive compensation for affiliating with or being employed by a firm, partnership, association, corporation, or other entity providing professional services involved in any fiduciary relationship.*

- *Congressional member's names by a firm, partnership, association, corporation, or any entity involved in practicing a profession cannot be involved in a fiduciary relationship.*

- *Congressional members may not serve as a board member or an officer in any non-congressional corporation, association, or other entity.*

  Note: This membership restriction was intended to include the <u>American Legislative Exchange Council, (ALEC)</u>, and the <u>Trilateral Commission, (TC)</u>, which are both very well organized national and international consortiums of current and previous federal and state politicians and powerful international corporations involving thousands of members. They claim to be non-partisan public-private partnerships with both federal and state governments — however they are lobbying to increase corporate profits at public expense. Of the 104 members of ALEC who <u>are active politicians</u>, 10 were active Republican Senators, while only one member is a Democrat. And of some 64 active Republicans from the House of Representatives, only one is Democrat. Of the 30 members that were previously members of the House, 29 are Republican, and only one is a Democrat. Both ALEC and TC serve as government consultants and lobbyists, creating self-serving Bills that use they're own federal and state legislative members to jointly prepare policies that powerful corporations and their lobbyists and special interest members have prepared for current state and federal House and Senate members to approve later <u>as written</u>. ALEC drafts and proposes legislation for each state, bringing together international corporations and their partisan Republican legislators to write and propose a variety of bills — many dealing with gun laws, voter suppression, union-busting policies — as well as a whole series of self-serving and controversial legislation. ALEC's national network of state and federal politicians and powerful corporations is designed solely to increase corporate profits without ever being scrutinized by the public. Does this sound like a democracy of the people?

- *A member may not teach without prior notification to and approval of the Senate Select Committee on Ethics for Senators, or the House Committee on Standards of Official Conduct for the House of Representatives.*

- *Members of the House of Representatives and Senators cannot accept honoraria. Outside Earned Income means, wages, salaries, fees, and other amounts received as compensation for personal services rendered. The honoraria do not, however, include copyright royalties, received from established publishers under usual and customary contractual terms.*

Tax Deductions:
Tax deductions allow members to deduct from income tax their living expenses up to $3,000 per annum, while away from their congressional districts or home states.

The Senators' Official Personnel and Office Expense Account (SOPOEA):
The SOPOEA expense account pays from $2,361,820 for a Senator representing a state with a population under 5 million to $3,753,614 for a Senator representing a state with a population of more than 28 million.

Other Salaries and Allowances and Congressional Research Service:
Shows a range of $2,960,726 to $4,685,279 depending on the state and the average allocation is $3,206,825. Members of Congress create their own very comprehensive single prepayment type Government Healthcare and Retirement benefits. However, *"We the People"* have unknowingly condoned this situation. What's even worse is these self-serving members spend far too much time administering their programs as well as constantly seeking re-election donations, therefore having little or almost no time to deal with their full-time job or the very serious major issues confronting this nation. On top of all this, Congressmen are constantly ping-ponging the other party's policies they've accomplished, while forgetting what "We the People," that hire them, want. In fact, the House and Senate have made fewer and fewer decisions that have helped the country during the last three President's terms, and now they can't even approve the nation's annual fiscal budget promptly. Why? — Because they are so busy politicizing their party's liberal or conservative views and seeking donations they've forgotten who they represent.

The following analysis of the 100 Federal Senators by region, is far more cost-effective than the 435 members of the House but could be reduced to one Senator per state.

Current Senate (#100)

Region	States and Senate Seats	Population	Seat Ratio /Senate
New England	MA-2, CT-2, ME-2, NH-2, RI-2, VT-2 #(12)	14,618,806	1/1,193,689
Mid Atlantic	MA-2, CT-2, ME-2, NH-2, RI-2, VT-2 #(6)	41,324,267	1/6,887,378
S. Atlantic	FL-2, GA-2, NC-2, VA-2, MD-2, SC-2, WV-2, DE-2, DC #(16)	61,783,647	1/3,861,478
E.S. Central	TN-2, AL-2, KY-2, MS-2 #(8)	18,716,202	1/2,339,525
W.S. Central	TX-2, LA-2, OK-2, AR-2 #(8)	37,883,604	1/4,735,450
E.N. Central	IL-2, OH-2, MI-2, IN-2, WI-2 #(10)	46,662,180	1/4,666,218
W.N. Central	MO-2, MN-2, IA-2, KS-2, NE-2, SD-2, ND-2 #(14)	20,885,710	1/1,491,836
Mountain	AZ-2, CO-2, UT-2, NV-2, NM-2, ID-2, MT-2, WY-2 #(16)	22,881,245	1/1,430,078
Pacific	CA-2, WA-2, OR-2, HI-2, AK-2 #(10)	51,373,178	1/5,137,318

Current House of Representatives (#435)

Region	States & House Seats	Population	Seat Ratio / Rep.
New England	MA, 9 CT, 5 ME, 2 NH, 2 RI, 2 VT 1 #(21)	14,618,806	1/696,134
Mid Atlantic	NY, 27 PA, 18 NJ #(57)	41,324,267	1/724,987
S. Atlantic	FL,27 GA,14 NC,13 VA,11 MD,8 SC,7 WV,3 DE,1 DC,1 #(85)	61,783,647	1/726,826
E.S. Central	TN, 9 AL, 7 KY, 6 MS 4 #(26)	18,716,202	1/719,853
W.S. Central	TX, 36 LA, 6 OK, 5 AR 9 #(56)	37,883,604	1/676,493
E.N. Central	IL, 18 OH, 16 MI, 14 IN, 9 WI 8 #(65)	46,662,180	1/717,880
W.N. Central	MO, 8 MN, 8 IA, 4 KS, 4 NE, 3 SD, 1 ND #(29)	20,885,710	1/720197
Mountain	AZ,9 CO,7 UT,4 NV,4 NM,3 ID,2 MT,1 WY,1 #(31)	22,881,245	1/789,008
Pacific	CA,53 WA,10 OR,5 HI,2 AK 1 (#71)	53-10-5-2-1	1/723.566

In reviewing the Independent State's Legislative jobs, they vary by the states they serve. State legislative appointments are not a full-time job, and most elected officials in most states balance their public work with their day jobs and balance personal and public responsibilities as best they can. On top of this, they frequently attend special sessions. California hires full-time legislatures at $90,000/year, and New York and Pennsylvania also hire full-time state legislators, while New Hampshire pays its part-time lawmakers $200 for a two-year term. Alaska, Florida, Illinois, Massachusetts, Michigan, Ohio, and Wisconsin hire fewer full-time legislatures at $50,000 per year plus a per diem of $200.00 with an allowance for office expenses and staff. Twenty-four states pay legislatures the equivalent of two-thirds of their full-time job on state business. Montana, Nevada, North Dakota and Texas meet on a biannual basis, and the Texas Legislature holds 140-day legislative sessions bi-annually unless the governor calls a special session. The remaining 16 states operate on a part-time basis.

3

Elections

Popular Vote vs. Electoral College:
Elections have become the second greatest obstacle to the U.S. remaining a democracy that protects the equality of "We the People" — and this freedom will perish if the people do not strongly resist what's currently happening in the U.S. election process. In November of a presidential election year, each state holds an open election for all the qualified citizen voters to select their most popular choice for President and Vice-President — but what happens after their voting is not understood by most citizens. It is at this point that either the liberal or conservative party that receives most of the votes in a state can choose a slate of electors called the *"Electoral College"* who will cast their vote for President and Vice-President, ignoring the overall popular vote of the people. The United States has now had this current Multi-party "Winner Take All System" since 1876, under this double plurality voting where unsupervised political factions have had total control over the Popular Vote. George Washington ran as an Independent and was elected President three times from 1788 to 1792, and John Tyler and Andrew Jackson who had no major party affiliation also were elected President by the people. From 1829 to the end of the Civil War in 1856, the people's vote previously appointed Presidents from six independent political parties and those parties were the Democratic-Republican Party, the Federalist Party, the National Republican Party, the Whig Party and an earlier Republican type party. However, today's Multi-party system has taken over since 1876, and we the people now have to ask just who represents the people in today's Multi-party systems? Are we really *"a government of the people, by the people, for the people"*?

26

For example:

> *The election of 1876 pitted Samuel J. Tilden, the Democratic governor of New York, against Rutherford B. Hayes, the Republican governor of Ohio, which offers an example of how the people's vote has become so meaningless. It appeared that Tilden won the popular vote with 184 electoral votes to Hayes's 165 - however, 185 electoral votes were required, which made it necessary for the electoral commission to determine who would become president. Because of an unbalanced Republican Commission and five members of the non-political Supreme Court that openly voted along Republican party-lines, they selected Rutherford B. Hayes to become President. Because of this, the Democrats threatened to disrupt any orderly transfer of power to Hayes, but the Republicans agreed to withdraw the federal troops that still occupied the South following the end of the Civil War in 1865 — and to provide funds for the recovery of the largely Democratic South. They also agreed to appoint at least one Southerner to the cabinet, and in return, the Democrats agreed not to impede Hayes's inauguration, and so the people's popular vote meant nothing. Even today, the Supreme Court and the congressional Multi-party system ignores the people of each state.*

So, let's take a closer look at the parties that profess to represent "We the People."

The Libertarian Party (LP):

The LP promotes civil liberties, interventionism and laissez-faire capitalism and the abolition of the welfare state. The founding of the LP was due to the Vietnam War and the total discontinuance of the Gold standard under President Nixon. The LP promotes a classical liberal platform like the Republican conservative platform and the Democrats progressive and modern liberal platforms. They also promote policies that lower taxes and would eliminate the IRS that created this country's first income tax in 1913, which had previously been declared unconstitutional by the Supreme Court in 1895. However, in 1913, it seemed reasonable enough to pay income tax on only one percent of income under $20,000, with the assurance that it would never increase — which never happened. The LP would also seek to decrease the national debt that in 2016 was $18.96 trillion, and allowed people to get out of Social Security; eliminate welfare by promoting private charities; prohibit illegal drugs; promote gun ownership; support same-sex marriages, and lower the drinking age to 18.

The Green Party:

The Green Party is a formally organized political third-party based on the principles of social justice, environmentalism and nonviolence, which provides a foundation for world peace through its international Global Green Organization. Green party platforms typically embrace social-democratic economic policies and the promotion of coalitions with the leftists.

The Constitution Party:

The constitution party is a national third-party who basis their platform on their interpretations of the U.S. Constitution, the principles of the Declaration of Independence and the Bible.

All third parties have little chance of forming a government or winning the position of President, but there are many reasons for third parties to compete because they help expand the vision beyond Congresses' sole attention to just the Liberal or Conservative factions.

Today's Electoral College gets one electoral vote for each member of its House of Representatives, based on the state's population and the two votes for each state Senator. With all the problems the U.S. is having with today's Multi-party system, there is little question that a popular vote would make the election process substantially more democratic, but doing that requires the U. S. to amend the Constitution. Every state, including the District of Columbia, has been given at least a minimum of three electoral votes regardless of the size of their population to better represent the smaller states than if they were recognized solely by their population. However, this has also resulted in the overall distribution of Electoral College votes per state to no longer be equally dispersed based on population. When the total number of votes are counted based on the number of Senate and House members, with a minimum of 3 votes for all states and the District of Columbia, there are some 538 Senate and House Electors that comprise the Electoral College. The College members then meet at a designated location within their respective state in December to cast the official ballot for the President and Vice-President, thereby appointing the candidate who receives a majority of the Electoral College's votes (currently 270) which wins the election. What's so frightening about this Electoral College system of voting is it renders the popular vote useless, which is not understood or accepted by most of the citizens of the United States and because of this it makes the people feel their vote is unimportant. CNN indicated that voter turnout in 2016 dipped to nearly its lowest point in two decades. And although election officials were still tabulating ballots in June 2017, the 126 million votes previously counted show that only 55% of voting age citizens cast ballots that year. That measure of turnout is the lowest in a presidential election since 1996 when 53.5% of voting-age citizens turned out. So why vote? Losing control of the people's voice in the U.S. elections is directly attributable to the power of today's Multi-party system once again taking control over what was once a single party representing the people during the "Era of Good Feelings" from 1829 to 1850 when partisan politics resurfaced. In the last three presidential terms, this Multi-party system overruled the popular vote twice. Al Gore won 48.4% of the popular vote in the 2000 election, while George W. Bush, received 47.9%. However, the Electoral College's two-party system and the Supreme Court awarded G. W. Bush 271 Electoral Votes while former Vice-President Gore received 266. And now, in the 2016 election, Hillary Clinton received 65,844,610 popular votes, or 48.2%, which totaled 2.86 million more popular votes than D. Trump, and yet — the Electoral College awarded Donald Trump the Presidency after he received 62,979,636 or 46.1% of the popular votes. This imbalance between the Electoral College and the popular vote is now happening almost every election year, and it's time the U.S. amend the Constitution to remove the failing Electoral College system's control of this nation's elections.

2016 – 538 Total Electoral Votes:

3 Electoral Votes –Population

Alaska	735,132
Delaware	925,749
District of Columbia	646,449
Montana	1,015,165
North Dakota	723,393
South Dakota	844,877
Vermont	626,630
Wyoming	582,658

4 Electoral Votes –Population

Hawaii	1,404,054
Idaho	1,612,136
Maine	1,328,302
New Hampshire	1,323,459
Rhode Island	1,051,511

5 Electoral Votes –Population

Nebraska	1,868,516
New Mexico	2,085.287
West Virginia	1,854,304

6 Electoral Votes –Population

Arkansas	2,959,373
Iowa	3,090,416
Kansas	2,893,957
Mississippi	2,991,207
Nevada	2,790,136
Utah	2,900,872

7 Electoral Votes –Population

Connecticut	3,596,080
Oklahoma	3,850,568
Oregon	3,930,065

8 Electoral Votes –Population

Kentucky	4,395,295
Louisiana	4,625,470

9 Electoral Votes –Population

Alabama	4,833,722
Colorado	5,268,367
South Carolina	4,774,839

10 Electoral Votes –Population

Maryland	5,928,814
Minnesota	5,420,380
Missouri	6,044,171
Wisconsin	5,742,713

11 Electoral Votes –Population
Arizona	6.626,624
Indiana	6,570,902
Massachusetts	6,692,824
Tennessee	6,495,978

12 Electoral Votes –Population
Washington	6,971,406

13 Electoral Votes –Population
Virginia	8,260,405

14 Electoral Votes –Population
New Jersey	8,899,339

15 Electoral Votes –Population
North Carolina	9,848,060

16 Electoral Votes –Population
Georgia	9,992,167
Michigan	9,895,622

18 Electoral Votes –Population
Ohio	11,570,808

20 Electoral Votes –Population
Illinois	12,882,135
Pennsylvania	12,773,801

29 Electoral Votes –Population
Florida	19,552,860
New York	19,651,127

38 Electoral Votes –Population
Texas	26,448.193

55 Electoral Votes –Population
California	38,332,521

The above chart outlined this information to point out how different the size of the playing field has become under these two bicameral separate lawmaking assemblies. Let's also review how some states have become either *"Swing States"* or *"Safe States."* Swing States have maintained equal support for the candidates of either party in the past, while the Safe States are where the state always votes in favor of either a Democrat or a Republican. Texas, Arizona, Georgia, Tennessee, and Indiana, are "the Safe States" for Republicans and as a result, every Democrat's vote in these states becomes worthless. New York, California, Maryland, Illinois, Washington, and a few other variable states have historically been the Safe States for Democrats — while Swing states include Colorado, Florida, Ohio, New Hampshire, Virginia, Iowa, Maine, Michigan, Minnesota, Nevada, North Carolina, Pennsylvania, and Wisconsin. However, if you are a resident of a Swing State, say Florida for example, your vote is marginally more significant than the vote of an individual in a Safe State. Therefore, if a candidate wins the popular vote of a state by just one vote, that candidate receives all the electoral votes of that state (excluding Maine and Nebraska). Should the opinion of one person over-write the will of thousands or even millions of American voters?

Texas, a Safe Republican State, is where the Republican Congress received thirty-eight (38) electoral votes in 2016. The imbalance of the take all Electoral College votes, versus not splitting the popular vote of 26,448,193 million Texas votes won the election for the Republican candidate. Another imbalance in this Multi-party system involves the smaller states like Wyoming where they received one electoral vote for every 194,289 people based on a total population of 582,658, providing 3.6 electoral votes in Wyoming for every single vote in Texas. In Texas, where the playing field favors the Multi-party system over the single popular vote, it takes 696,005 people to receive one vote — suggesting there is no way to beat the winner take all concept of the Electoral College. The Electoral College is a ridiculous concept that allows today's Multi-party congress to control the people's elections. Worse yet — the U.S. democracy is far too often finding itself playing on an unlevel playing field where the citizen's majority vote only determines which candidate will receive all the electoral votes, while the popular vote does not count as a direct vote for the President. And now with the Russian cyber-attack disrupting this nation's elections, Americans can only wonder if the U.S. is still a democracy.

Since only 55% of the eligible voters voted in 2016, and almost half of those voters were Democrats and half were Republicans — it suggests that only one-quarter of the total population appointed the president rather than the entire voter population under a populist voting system. In fact, one need no longer wonder why the U.S. voter has lost interest in trying to elect a President to this most important office in the world.

The Electoral College appointees that vote against the will of the people in a state are called *"Faithless Electors."* Although these congressionally appointed electors are usually extremely loyal to the party they align with; they don't have to vote the way the popular vote instructed them. Nor just because a candidate won the popular vote in a state, it does not mean these congressionally appointed electors can't cast a vote for the people's candidate. Twenty-nine states have legislation that penalizes Faithless Electors, but these states have never penalized any voter that didn't vote with their party, while twenty-one states do not mandate that an elector must vote for his or her party's candidate. Electing a President by the popular vote holds far more weight and significance than a political party's "take all system." Under a people's system, each citizen would be voting for President, and no longer under the control of some powerful, wealthy international corporate voter.

Although campaign debates are to allow the people to see and evaluate the candidates in person, the current *"mud-slinging contests"* have only proven to be detrimental and of no value when they become contests that only play the *"blame-game."* Debates should more appropriately be discussions about what the candidate propose to do if elected to become President, Senator, or a member of the House of Representatives. Today, these candidates are far more concerned with shooting arrows at other candidates or the Republican or Democratic Party than clearly stating why they are qualified to achieve their plan of accomplishment or how they intend to finance the goals and objectives they propose for public review before the election. Every candidate should be required to prepare their resume just as they do with any job application for the public to read and evaluate. But more importantly, they should be required to present a written *"Plan of Accomplishment"* so the public can later measure their actual success once they have served in office. The public would also be far better prepared to elect the most qualified candidate based on the best professionally presented *"Plan of Accomplishment"* — rather than demeaning one another for an hour and a half or more at some mud-slinging contest. Democrats are criticizing Republicans and Republicans are damning every Democrat, and this eventually leads to destroying any relationship that's required when they do serve in office and need to bilaterally pass laws, rules, regulations, and policies, or propose amendments that benefit the people. Based on today's degrading debates between Republican and Democratic parties, is it any wonder why we have a dysfunctional and confused House of Representatives and Senate — which is in continuous conflict because of the ridiculous Multi-party's lack of interest in representing we the people?

Following World War II, the U.S. Congress' Multi-party was primarily nonpartisan, not taking either liberal or conservative sides, and often providing bipartisan support in solving problems. However, in the mid-sixties, political polarization began to increase as wealthy corporate financial donations began to influence some of the political party members on selected issues such as health insurance and the cost of pharmaceutical drugs. These issues presented a problem for Congress because of the wealthy faction's McCarran Ferguson Act that allowed profit seekers to earn money from the sick and disabled while being asked to approve Medicare and Medicaid. As a result, the Multi-party Congress began to use partisanship tactics on issues they'd previously compromised on, such as the private non-profit Blue Cross Blue Shield noninsurance healthcare prepayment program. However, once the powerful outside marketing factions were able to influence Congress, the Republicans saw this as a potential source of additional payback for favors, and they supported profit insurance that became the only health care coverage system in the entire world that sought a profit from the sick and disabled. As a result, in the seventies and eighties, political gridlock began to take place, and the Multi-party Congress had far more difficulty passing bills and laws that satisfied the agenda of the people's democracy — and this has now brought this nation to a political standstill. Today's Republican *"Party of Power"* now involves the executive branch of government, which in the past has served as a neutral autonomous political power that brought the Congress together. In 1979, former President Gerald Ford while speaking to healthcare officials discussed the importance of every President *"Balancing the Iron Cross"* — which had long been an important requirement for every President. Balancing the Iron Cross required every President try to maintain a fair and just balance between the four ends of the cross that represented the *"People,"* the *"Politicians,"* the *"Lobbyist and Bureaucracy,"* and the *"Armed Services."* Shockingly, in the year 2000, the "Sacrosanct" Supreme Court also inadvertently became involved in this political balancing act as a fifth appendage when they politically (not legally) appointed the Republican Presidential candidate to the White House in a bitter bipartisan battle. The Presidential office was obligated to try and resolve the growing number of Multi-party liberal and conservative issues that were causing the Senate and House of Representatives to become so dysfunctional. In addition to the Iron Cross obligations, it is now also becoming blatantly apparent that the Congress is ignoring the presidential candidate's personal, financial, and credential qualifications as they blindly sanction far too many unqualified candidates for the position of the President of the United States — one of the most important offices in the world.

Being strongly *"Partisan"* involves a committed member of a Congressional Multi-party that refuses to compromise with their political opponents by staunchly favoring their party, which constitutes *"Illegal Partisan Extremism,"* and violates the U.S. Constitution. The Republican Party recently met behind closed doors to attempt to pass a new healthcare Act in secret, which constituted *"Illegal Partisan Extremism."* By attempting to pass their Healthcare Bill without bipartisan involvement promotes a Dictatorship rather than a Democracy.

The Congress has also failed to annually approve the fiscal budget, which is beyond belief when in 2018, the U.S. has an $18,596 billion deficit in the GDP.

> *The national debt of the United States is the amount owed (Deficit) by the federal government of the United States. The measure of the public debt is the value of the outstanding Treasury securities at the point of time issued by the Treasury and other federal government agencies.*

> *The <u>Gross Domestic Product (GDP)</u> in the United States was worth 18036.65*

billion US dollars in 2015. The GDP value of the United States represents 29.09 percent of the world economy. GDP in the United States averaged 6560.26 USD Billion from 1960 until 2015, reaching an all-time high of 18036.65 USD Billion in 2015 and a record low of 543.30 USD Billion in 1960.

4

Healthcare

"We the People" need to understand this nation's freedom may soon perish if the people do not strongly resist what's been happening to this nation's healthcare tax benefit since 1960, a result of the profit-seeking *"McCarran-Ferguson Act,"* passed in 1945. Profit-seeking in a human service to humanity has become a very chronic problem in the U.S., the only country in the world that does not protect the earned benefits of its people equally.

History:
Let's briefly review the history of medicine just before the twentieth century, which should help to demonstrate how medical and cultural systems once fostered medicine as an *"Art Form"* rather than a true science based on shared democratic principles and the rule of law.

Changing this deeply entrenched art form of the nineteenth-century required the U.S. first recognize, understand, and deal with the *"Witch Doctor Syndrome"* that attempted to cure sickness and exorcise evil spirits by the use of religious rituals, magic, witchcraft, voodoo, and secret potions rather than scientific medical necessity. Religious beliefs, superstition, and fear of the unknown that protected the Witch Doctor from any form of scrutiny — allowed tribe members to assume almost no responsibility for their well-being. As healthcare advanced into the 1890s, it included various trades or guilds of practitioners such as midwives, herbalists, compounders, bone setters, barber-surgeons, and numerous other artisans. Each trade practiced with a certain body of knowledge, such as the barber-surgeon who tended baths, cut hair, pulled teeth, lanced boils, and bled and purged the circulatory system that supposedly eliminated disease or infection from the body. The red, white, and blue barber pole that identifies today's barbershop served as the barber surgeon's symbol — representing the white bandage, the blue venous blood, and the red arterial blood.

Hospitals in the early twentieth-century were nothing more than dumping places for wounded soldiers, the epidemic diseased, and the poor, while the wealthy received care in their homes, usually by the most qualified practitioner available. Hospitals were where patients went to die, which were referred to as *"Pest Houses"* because they dealt primarily with epidemics and contagious diseases. Hospital sanitation was unheard of as patients went unbathed and hospital bed linens seldom changed. Worse yet, in times of epidemic disease, beds were not available. Surgery was also a torturous procedure with no anesthesia and involved a very high risk of infection, which consisted almost entirely of amputations and gangrenous wounds. The infections bred in hospitals killed more patients than the original diseases or injuries. Even up to the 1930s, when patients were required to go to the hospital, they far too often resigned themselves to die there.

In the Crimean War of 1853, Florence Nightingale converted an army barracks into the first hospital at Scutari on the other side of the Straits of Constantinople. At this hospital, she reduced the mortality rate from 60 percent to less than 1 percent by providing the sick or injured with light, fresh air, cleanliness, warmth, and nutrition. She spent hours with dying soldiers bringing light and warmth to the bedside for which she became known as the "Lady with the Lamp" and the "Angel of Crimea," — and she believed that by improving the surroundings nature would heal, which probably was the best advice medicine ever received. Her efforts later resulted in clean beds, sanitary surroundings, proper nutrition, and qualified nurses in many of the hospitals by the 1930s. She constantly wrote, publishing *"Notes on Nursing"* in 1860, before she became ill and lived in a sick room until she died at 90 years of age, on August 13, 1910. She attempted to take the power of nursing out of the hands of the often-maligned politician, community leaders and untrained practitioners, which also identified her as the "Rebel with a Cause" — a battle that intensified today with corporate profit-seekers in Washington D.C. Her writings and consultation played an important role in establishing the first nursing training schools in the United States.

Massachusetts was the first state in the U.S. to attempt to define a medical education by issuing a license to Harvard students that received a regular college diploma or passed a qualifying medical examination. By 1875, some forty-seven schools provided diplomas to college graduates that sought to practice medicine even though they did not complete a defined medical curriculum. And worse yet, these licensed practitioners who sought to set educational standards were aggressively opposed by a majority of practitioners that still resisted any regulation at all. By 1885, there were close to 500 undefined programs attempting to graduate a variety of undereducated and ill-trained medical practitioners, which is a characteristic we still accept today when patients seek the services of a physician without investigating the physician's previous training or preparation. In fact, before 1910, very few medical school standards had any substance to them, providing only a license to live under the college's name. Most of the colleges that provided these programs were public service corporations supported by taxation or private endowment, but far too many consumers were unaware that physician's credentials were nonexistent.

All this medical chaos finally began to yield during the first thirty years of the twentieth-century when anesthesia, radiology, antisepsis, and the germ theory of disease first began to be practiced in the healthcare field. So after nineteen centuries of inadequate healthcare, Nightingale, Roentgen, and Pasteur's scientific achievements finally began to replace the many *"Art Forms"* that had previously involved religious rituals, magic, witchcraft, voodoo, and secret potions with new understandable scientific procedures. But this also had a downside in that these scientific advancements were beginning to show that medicine was far more complex than the medieval cults or trade schools had realized, and proper educational training became an obvious need as science began to expose the complex network of systems that comprised the human body. The previous practitioners also no longer could remain all-knowing regarding the circulatory system; the nervous system; the respiratory system; the musculoskeletal system; the digestive system; the immune system; the endocrine system; infectious and genetic diseases; clinical procedures;

pharmaceuticals; and the hundreds of other related medical complexities. As a result, the federal government, the states, and the communities and philanthropic organizations all began to take the initial steps to protect the individual patient's rights by defining healthcare's *"Shared Principles and the Rule of Law"* — however, nineteen centuries of suppression and control was not to end easily. That was until educational standards were initially defined in the 1910 *"Flexner Report"* by the Carnegie and Rockefeller Foundations — which pointed up many serious conditions that were referred to as *"Scandalous"* — while recommending that all patients should receive care from properly trained physicians. The Flexner Report was responsible for establishing proper licensing of trained and qualified physicians that took the *"Hippocratic Oath of Do No Harm"* after completing an approved medical education curriculum with defined medical standards.

It wasn't until 1907, when "Typhoid Mary," (Mary Mallon) was taken into custody by quarantine by the New York City Health Department, who estimated she caused at least three deaths by typhoid fever. However, estimates suggest she may have caused as many as 50 fatalities. Mallon was the first asymptomatic or healthy typhoid carrier identified, and there were no policies or guidelines for the handling of such a problem, and she declined to acknowledge any connection between her cooking and the typhoid cases by saying she never had typhoid fever. Other asymptomatic typhoid carriers identified in the early twentieth-century were: Tony Labella, who allegedly caused as many as 100 cases and five deaths; "Typhoid John," who it was estimated to have infected 36 people and caused two deaths; and Alphonse Cotils along with several hundred other healthy-carriers were finally properly isolated. However, it wasn't until August 1913, when medicine was finally able to successfully identify the many asymptomatic carriers who contaminated food and water, realizing that a human carrier was usually a healthy person who experienced an episode of typhoid fever and then continued to shed the bacteria through their feces or urine. Washing hands, dishes and utensils with soap and water, and not eating or drinking contaminated food or water then became the ways one could reduce the risk of becoming infected with typhoid.

Blue Cross incorporated in 1929, and Blue Shield in 1939, forming BCBS. BCBS became a very successful privately-owned *nonprofit-noninsurance* pre-payment program that paid no taxes and was regulated by each state as a *"Community Rated System"* — meaning everyone paid the same rate for their healthcare regardless of age, sex, where they lived, or how sick they were. Next, in 1946, the *"Hill-Burton Hospital Survey and Construction Act"* provided federal grants that guaranteed loans to improve this country's nonprofit hospitals, which became one of the first healthcare government programs formed to help meet the hospital growth demands from two previous world wars. The government used tax dollars to accomplish a 4.5-bed ratio per a 1,000 population for the hospitals, which were all non-profit, and which were not allowed to discriminate based on race, color, national origin, or creed while being required to provide a reasonable amount of uncompensated care for twenty years.

Then in 1945, Congress, in direct opposition to these tax-supported non-profit hospitals, shockingly passed the *"McCarran-Ferguson Act,"* opening the door to competitive profit-seeking insurance prepayment healthcare, which later in the early '60s spiraled healthcare costs out of control by adding an insurance profit to this country's cost of health care. As a result, the U.S. became the only country in the world, seeking to profit from their sick and disabled. In 1965 President Johnson recommended that Congress pass *Medicare* and *Medicaid* because of the high cost of healthcare, in an attempt to replace the costly McCarran-Ferguson transgression. Medicare provided health coverage for those who were 65 or older or had a severe disability — and Medicaid, which is a state and federal program providing health coverage for those with a very low income. Because of public dissatisfaction with profit-seeking insurance, the Congress chose to return to partner with BCBS to administer Medicare, while selfishly and secretly creating a special *"Federal Employees Health Benefits Program"* (FEHB) for themselves and all Federal Employees. If only the FEHB government program could have at that time become a single nonprofit program for the Armed Services, the VA, and the Public, the U.S. would have had far fewer problems today. Then in the early '60s, just when things were seriously trending back to a single prepayment program, profit insurance and the Pharmaceutical industry labeled the people's government supported healthcare programs as *"Socialistic."* These wealthy factions also aggressively lobbied Congress for favors, by providing substantial donations for the politician's re-election campaigns, which made far too many unethical politicians wealthy. These favors discouraged many of the politicians from ever returning to a single nonprofit cost-effective health care system — while the U.S. world healthcare ranking dropped from first in the world to thirty-seventh by the *World Health Organization (WHO)* and today to thirty-second. As profit insurance aggressively moved to take control of this country's cost-effective non-profit healthcare prepayment program, they began to pursue only healthy clients and working groups to buy cheaper *"Tiered (low-risk) Group Rated"* profit insurance. Profit insurance clients did not have a clue that each group rate would significantly increase costs as its members decreased in number due to pre-existing health-related problems and age. This reduction in number forced the "Blues" to cover more of the pre-existing conditions, the pregnant women, the aged, and the sick and disabled that profit insurance dumped by increasing their premiums to unrealistic levels that often reached several thousands of dollars a month.

In 2015, profit insurance premiums increased to 33% of the nation's 3.2 Trillion Dollar Annual Cost for Health Care, while Medicare increased 20% and Medicaid State and Federal increased 17%. The Veteran's Administration (VA) increased 4%, and the Affordable Care Act (ACA), as well as all the other costs and the out of pocket costs together, increased 27%. Due to party politics, current projections for ACA increases are falsely politicized, stating that their costs are spiraling out of control, which is not true. And it's now obvious that hospitals do not receive any trickle-down profits from profit insurance to improve patient's care. In fact, the hospitals of the 60's experienced huge financial losses as insurance profits spiraled healthcare costs out of control. As a result, hospitals were forced to develop *"Regional Planning* and *Cost Containment Programs."*

Previous Professional Research

Research became nationally recognized when it involved more than 5,000 volunteer doctors, nurses, and paraprofessionals in the 1960's who sought to cut the out of control costs of healthcare after Congress passed the 1945 McCarran-Ferguson Act. This Act opened the door to the profit-seekers and politicians in the mid 60's who ignored this voluntary professionally driven leading-edge research that sought to return health care to its number one ranking in the world, instead of 32nd. The Members of Congress ignored this research because they had found a way of lining their pockets with insurance and pharmaceutical kickbacks for favors. Ignoring the addition of this huge profit margin that was added to the cost of healthcare, this group of healthcare professionals determined that the hospital's de-centralized paper medical record system was also causing much of the costly inefficiencies in health care. Their research determined the medical record was comprised of about 375 different forms, although some larger hospitals had as many as 1,600 separate and distinct medical record forms. These manual forms were not standardized and were very costly to print, file, and maintain in a manual system that was decentralized and not able to make universal patient medical record information readily available — aside from not being very confidential. It was embarrassing to find that America's automobile manufacturers, electricians, and plumbers, had far better standards for consumer protection than healthcare in the United States. In that the primary ownership and legal rights to a patient's medical record belonged to the patient, these decentralized manual facility records were seldom if ever readily available to the patient in this maze of decentralized multiple healthcare facilities. If the U.S. continues to develop the current ridiculous manual system or tries to computerize this decentralized system, things will take longer and become far more costly and confused — thereby only delaying the patient from ever obtain any accountability for their clinical well-being. As a result, these researchers suggested that a community-based computer network of patient-owned healthcare information offered the best solution to this nation's current medical record. After completing a single "community" patient record, a nationwide database network could next be accomplished — setting national standards and laws so a patient or their designate could obtain legal access to their total health record and assume greater responsibility for there own well-being

These professional volunteers determined that comprehensive healthcare in the United States also needed a professionally stable non-profit single health care prepayment service led by professionally trained health care providers that abide by the Hippocratic Oath, not politicians that seek financial kickbacks. In fact, the current Multi-party U.S. political systems have been "Ping – Ponging" health care from nonprofit to profiting from the sick and disabled since 1965, depending on which Congressional party is in power. The U.S. can no longer allow healthcare in America to continue under the conservative and liberal parties that continuously flip-flop the unnecessary spiraling healthcare costs totally out of control. Nor can this nation remain the only nation in the world that has no human compassion for its citizens as profit insurance and the pharmaceutical industry, and a select group of opportunistic Congressmen seeks to profit from this nation's tax-paying sick and disabled.

"We the People" need a single comprehensive healthcare noninsurance prepayment program under a single non-profit private and government tax-supported program that is both a tax supported benefit and a right for every citizen. Also combining the following programs into a single nonprofit program will help to additionally reduce the spiraling costs of healthcare in the U.S. — which should include all of the following:

   The Armed Services Healthcare Systems
   The Veteran's Administration Systems (VA)
   The Federal Employees and Politicians Health Benefits Program
   (FEHB),
   The Medicare/Medicaid and the Affordable Care Act (ACA) and all
   of Child Care and all profit-seeking insurance programs

The patient or their designate should also be able to readily obtain online access to their total clinical database at any approved online location. This research determined that the security to this single comprehensive system needed to be well defined, approved, and professionally protected and maintained before a comprehensive, cost-effective national network could ever become viable. This research will also be a huge undertaking that requires continued financial tax support and involvement and is every bit as big and important as the space shots this nation has already paid for and accomplished. These professionals evaluating and defining these future concepts have confirmed that the consumer will someday demand and understand the importance of these types of improvements to stop the unmanageable and non-confidential chaos that currently is tolerated by so many trusting patients. A confidential patient database will not only advance and significantly improve comprehensive patient care and treatment, but it will put an immediate end to the current misuse of private patient information. The installation of such a system will be costly upfront but will significantly cut healthcare costs dramatically when fully implemented. However, this type of system will require healthcare professionals to be allowed to assume overall responsibility, which excludes unqualified politicians and profit seekers from disrupting this nation's future healthcare system.

The Future Healthcare System:

A legally confidential database will permit critical analysis, evaluation, and measurement of the quality of patient care without ever exposing the patient's or doctor's identity unless required. The computer is far more capable of imposing far greater confidentiality standards than today's decentralized manual and disorganized computer maze of paper confusion that allows almost any hospital or insurance employee to read a patient's confidential record. It is also important to realize that medicine is desperately in need of regaining their professional leadership in designing a comprehensive healthcare *"database"* network. Some of today's partial computer systems have helped the patient communicate with the doctor by reviewing reports and scheduling appointments and ordering drugs, but healthcare must next take the much larger step toward a single confidential and comprehensive patient medical record database that is owned by and readily available to the patient. This single medical record will also allow only authorized qualified health professionals to measure and audit clinical performance accurately and confidentially. This system must automatically set basic clinical standards that help regulate, monitor, audit, and even suggests alternatives in assisting with the individual judgment and evaluation of every type of clinical disease and treatment in every type of healthcare facility. The health professionals must play a leadership role in setting, maintaining, and controlling the health record's confidentiality and standards, and they should not have to act as a clerk or typist when using the system. Providing an adequate patient database will benefit healthcare as a whole and will help reduce malpractice, injury, improper treatment, unnecessary tests and exams, and poor patient care.

Today's manual medical record coding is under a unitized terminal-digit numbering system, which only permits one patient's multiple paper medical records to be available under that patient's name or number in one specific facility. An interpretable comprehensive, cumulative, family unit numbering system for multiple facilities remains a dream for the future. Under a new family unit numbering system, anticipating that the human genome map will soon decipher the chemical book of life for related humans, a single record — identifying highly confidential patient and family heredity characteristics and DNA data will play a major part in the future comprehensive healthcare treatment regime. The identifying coding of the future will require a universal family unit database number for each patient. Standard diagnostic workups, with a problem and symptom library that directs or guides the physician to a list of prospective diagnoses or differential diagnoses, have not yet been implemented. Because of this, orders for a diagnostic workup or the treatment of a defined diagnosis cannot be dynamically monitored to determine either the treatment regimen or the success ratio. Accurate, dynamic, computer-based health record statistics on treatment procedures, diseases, deaths, complications, infections, function, etiology, topography, or heredity by geographic location all need to be dynamically made available for comprehensive patient treatment, education, audit, and planning. Accurate universal patient database statistics will be essential if health education and preventive care are ever to be effectively advanced. Patient database tools and diagnostic assistance are long overdue in today's decentralized manual-system, which far too often professes dishonestly to provide the best health care in the world. The U.S. was once ranked first in the world and now is at 32nd.

Recommended Healthcare Computer Equipment:
The history of the special *"Touch Sensitive Terminal"* that healthcare professionals researched and had manufactured provided the essential health professional human interface that used transaction concepts that can be readily interpreted by healthcare professionals. This terminal initiated revolutionary modifications to today's programming of the nine medical record applications that included the Patient Registration; History; Physical Examination; Problem List (DX); Progress Notes; Observations; Comparative Flow Charts; Updates; and Physician's Orders.

William C. Norris, President of Control Data Corporation (CDC) volunteered to provide the necessary computer confidential capability online and assigned Richard Dobrovolnay, their technical engineer, to come up with a terminal solution that didn't require nurses and doctors to perform clerical typing tasks. His solution was to apply a thin coating of

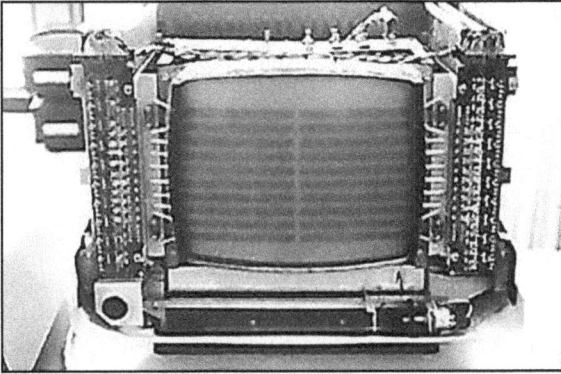

tin oxide mixed in a transparent solution of glue that's applied on a plastic sheet in two columns of ten lines on each side of what was to become the future CRT screen. By touching the appropriate line, the positive body-ion on one's finger completed the electronic circuit, switching the CRT. This selection of a complete *"transaction"* of words located behind a strip of clear glue and tin oxide on the face of the CRT (as shown here) became known as a *"transaction-oriented-entry."* As a result, the user's logical thought process controlled the sequential organization of each group of words desired for programming each application. The first Touch Sensitive Terminal was called the "Digiscribe," which was tested by over three-hundred physicians, nurses, educators, and paraprofessionals that all confirmed the unanimous acceptance of the touch-sensitive terminal as a very acceptable human interface to the professional end user who usually types poorly and does not wish to waste their valuable time performing disorganized clerical entries.

In 1969, the Department of Health and Welfare financed a study conducted by the Lockheed Company under contract PH 110-68-47 – Report No. LMSC 682084 National Center for Health Services Research and Development Dept. of H.E.W. entitled *"Analysis of Information Needs of Nursing Stations."* This study reported this was *"a system that will be far-reaching"* and that *"the nurses were very pleased with the Digiscribe."*

But no *"Computer Operating Systems (OS)* capable of handling a national database system was available in the early 1970s, which was a very big problem. However, in 1973, a new revolutionary Personal Computer (P.C.) system that when placed in tandem with a central operating system finally proved capable of handling the new bit mapping concept that allowed each bit of computer memory to control each CRT screen pixel, that utilized the subtle ramifications of touch and the use of standard screen template formats.

Screen formatting and entering structured transactions in a logical sequence, where the professional end user could design applications for programming was of course destined to have a major impact in reducing errors and correlating with the healthcare professional's thought process. These application display formatting standards revolutionized the end user design requirements by allowing health professionals to accomplish word display flowcharting, which is similar to architectural design before construction. User application designed flow charts were next adapted to plotters, simplifying the entire process of the professional healthcare user design. Another very important advantage of application formatting standards was the adaptability to Code Generation. These application designs eventually resulted in over 80% of the application programming being efficiently code generated by the computer, which exceeded previous efficient code generation by some 40%. At that time, Healthcare leaders had little knowledge that the Washington DC politicians strongly supported a decentralized healthcare system so they could continue their kickbacks for favors from a decentralized Pharmaceutical and Healthcare Insurance profit-seeking system. Congress and the many profit-seeking corporations that prefer decentralization so that they can profit from the enormous variety of decentralized healthcare systems have unknowingly destroyed any immediate hope for a single cost-effective nonprofit healthcare system. However, the people of this great Democracy will hopefully eventually realize that a universal, comprehensive national healthcare network will have a huge impact on the cost and quality of healthcare. Eventually the U.S. will be economically forced to accomplish a single paperless medical record as supported by President Ford when he said:

> *"To reduce the current out of control spiraling of health care costs, the current healthcare system will have to collapse."*

Perhaps then this nation's current rank of 32nd by the *"World Health Organization"* can once again be returned to the number one position it once held before the profit seekers invaded health care in the mid-1960s.

On May 5th, 2017, the U.S. Republican House voted 217 to 213 to place the cost of the *"Affordable Care Act (ACA),"* and some 45% of the state-funded *"Medicaid"* programs back on the people when their tax dollars previously paid for this. Fortunately, this proposal failed in the Senate even though a growing number of financially indigent citizens in the U.S. require this once tax paid human healthcare benefit for survival. This Republican closed-door (illegal) decision also attempted to boldly transfer more than 1.1 trillion dollars from healthcare to the .01% of billionaires (CFR) through tax reductions that were in total opposition to over eighty-five percent of the voting citizen's. More recently, the Republicans have not only voted to discontinue the ACA but perhaps parts of Medicare for thousands of citizens even though an overwhelming 85% of the population has opposed this repeal and replace bill of health care in America.

Eighty-five percent of the U.S. citizens feel one's tax dollars should provide health care as a "right" like every other country in the world. A tax-supported government program needs to stop this country's current totally out of control profiting from its sick and disabled. The 3.2 trillion dollars the U.S. is spending annually for health care is the most expensive in the world.

5

Budget and Finance

Based on this chapter's analysis of the U.S. budget, it suggests the citizen's immediately taking steps to recover the successful financial position the U.S. once held throughout the world. To accomplish this, Congress needs to agree to avoid all nongovernment congressional benefits and favors.

Signing the *"Norquist Pledge,"* which cannot even be printed without authorization — or becoming a member of the *"American Legislative Exchange Council (ALEC),"* clearly violates the congressman's Oath of Office. Some 238 Republican Members of the House and 41 Republican Senators, along with hundreds of state Republican officeholders have signed the Norquist Pledge of *"never to allow a tax increase"* as far back as 1990. This Norquist Pledge helped to cause today's tragic budget deficit that has significantly advanced Washington D.C.'s political gridlock. Recent surveys show that some 85% of *"We the People,"* and some 77% of the Republican voters think the Norquist Pledge was a bad idea. It does not take a *"Genius"* to understand that budgets require adjusting both income and expense either up or down annually by the start of the Fiscal Year, (October 1) and those that think otherwise are heading into troubled waters. Since the Clinton era had produced a $236 billion budget surplus, the George W. Bush 2000 White House felt it was acceptable to revise the United States tax-code by signing into law the following:

- The Economic Growth and Tax Relief Reconciliation Act (EGTRAA) of 2001.

- The Jobs and Growth Tax Relief Reconciliation Act (JGTRRA) of 2003.

- The Tax Relief, Unemployment Insurance Reauthorization, and Job Creation Act, became law in 2010.

These Tax Cuts had sunset provisions that made them expire at the end of 2010, but then they were foolishly extended for two years by President Barack Obama in 2010 — because the 2001 and 2003 Acts were incorrectly thought to have significantly reduced the tax rates for all U.S. taxpayers. However, a reduction was not the case, and there was a great deal of controversy as to who benefited from these tax cuts — or if they were effective in creating both jobs and meeting this nation's budgetary needs. The proponents of lower taxes argued that these tax cuts would increase the pace of this nation's economy and job growth even when the economy and job growth was not a major problem. The critics of the tax cuts said these tax cuts failed to encourage growth and would increase the budget deficit by shifting the tax burden from the rich to the middle class, which is what happened. These tax cuts seriously increased income inequality by shifting the tax burden away from the upper-income groups to the wage-earning households of the lower and middle class, while sky-rocketing the top 1%'s earnings to historical levels. The *"Alternative Minimum Tax (AMT),"* was a supplemental income tax imposed by the U.S. Federal Government in addition to the baseline income tax for certain individuals, corporations, estates, and trusts with exemptions or special circumstances that allowed for lower payments of standard income tax under the Internal Revenue Code. This ATM had not been adjusted to match the lowered Bush rates of the 2001 and 2003 Acts and was to end in 2017, but the 2001 and 2003 tax reductions had caused the middle-class wage earners to pay higher state and local taxes for themselves and their dependents as well as higher property taxes. The Internal Revenue Service tax-rate reductions for the top 0.1% of wage earners had been dropping from the year 1945 to 2005 from 60 % to 21%, and the top .01% had dropped from 55% to 24%. Because of the serious 2010 deficit, both of these wealthy categories were forced to adjust upward to 26% that year. The unemployment rate was 4% in 2000, increasing in 2003 to 6.1% and then to 10% by 2010 — which confirmed that the unemployment rate had increased without creating jobs because of these Bush Tax Cuts. And then when they reinstated the sunset provisions in the January 2013 tax year, there was finally a mandatory tax increase for the top 0.1% tax bracket back to 39.6% — close to where it was when this country had a budget surplus under the Clinton administration. When the United States returned to tax increases for the wealthy, the unemployment rate slowly started to decrease from 10 to 7.9 % according to the U.S. Bureau of Labor Statistics. The Bush tax cuts (EGTRRA and JGTRRA) had been the biggest cause of the 2008 depression as well as the current deficit, reducing revenues by about $1.8 trillion between 2002 and 2009. They also added close to $1.6 trillion to this country's debt between 2001 and 2011, excluding interest. The Democrats suggested that couples with incomes less than $250,000 not be subjected to any more tax increases. The Republicans sought to add the $3.3 trillion in loss of taxes to the national debt, and another $0.66 trillion for interest and debt service costs, pointing out the need for major tax policies that would never drive the U.S. back into the same problem in the future. If this nation ever intends to get the federal government back to making normal budget adjustments annually, it cannot allow partisan politicians to make decisions outside of normal budgetary analysis and adjustments based on experience. (Like decreasing the top wage earners tax so they can provide benefits to politicians that provide the wealthy faction financial favors.) On top of this, citizens now know that based on experience, the U.S. needs to increase current revenues substantially while decreasing spending by at least four trillion dollars over the next ten years. The Republican Majority, under the *"Norquist Pledge,"* has intentionally failed to approve timely annual budgets, which is beyond belief — and so the U.S. accumulated an $18.96 trillion gross national debt that will increase by at least ten trillion over the next ten years based on the current tax proposals. This time the Republicans are proposing cuts in the people's healthcare coverage so the conservatives can once again reduce the wealthy benefactors .01%'s tax burden — which in turn benefits the Congressmen who receive favors that never trickle down to the people. So let's review this country's depressions, recessions, panics, wars and the Presidents in charge during the entire twentieth century.

Twentieth-Century-Depressions-Recessions-Panics

Date of Depression (D) Recession NOW or Panic (P)	Dates	Duration	Peak Unem- ployed %	President R-Republican D- Democrat
R-1899-1900	6/99-12/00	1-Y-6-mo	5.0	T. Roosevelt- R
R-1902-1904	9/02- 8/04	1-Y-11-mo	4.8	T. Roosevelt- R
P-1907-1908	5/07-6/08	1-Y-1-mo	8.5	T. Roosevelt- R
P-1910-1912	1/10-1/12	2-Y	5.9	W. H. Taft- R
R-1013-1914	1/13-12/14	1-Y-11-mo	8.0	W. Wilson- D
R-19v18-1919	8/18-3/19	7-mo	2.3	W. Wilson- D
D-1920-1921	1/20-7/21	1-Y- 6-mo	11.9	W. Wilson- D
R-1923-1924	5/23- 6/24	1-Y- 2-mo	5.4	C. Coolidge- R
R-1926-1927	10/26-11/27	1-Y- 1-mo	4.1	C. Coolidge- R
D-1929-1933	8/29- 3/33	3-Y- 7-mo	24.9	H. Hoover- R
D-R-1933-1938	4/33- 6/38	5-Y-2-mo	21.7	F. D. Roosevelt- D
R-1945	2/45- 10/45	8-mo	1.9	F.D.R./H. Truman 4/21-D
R-1948- 1949	11/48-10/49	11-mo	6.6	H. S. Truman- D
R-1953- 1954	7/53-5/54	10-mo	4.5	D. D. Eisenhower- R
R-1957-1958	8/57- 4/58	8-mo	6.2	D. D. Eisenhower- R
R-1960-1961	4/60- 1/61	10-mo	6.6	D. D. Eisenhower- R
R-1969-1970	12/69-11/70	11-mo	6.1	R. M. Nixon- R
R-1973-1975	1/73- 3/75	1-Y- 4-mo	8.2	R. M. Nixon/G.R. Ford-R
R-1980	1/80- 7/80	6-mo	7.2	J. E. Carter- D
R-1981-1982	7/81- 11/82	1-Y- 4-mo	8.5	R. Reagan- R
R- 1990-1991	7/90- 3/91	8-mo	7.3	G. H. W. Bush- R
R- 2001	3/01- 11/01	8-mo	5.7	G. W. Bush- R
R-2007-2009	12/07 – 6/09	1- Y- 6-mo	9.9	G. W. Bush- R

There were 23 Depressions – Recessions or Panics from 1899 to 2009 of which 16 were while Republican Presidents were in office and six were while Democratic Presidents were in office. The Republicans had 251 months of Depressions, Recessions or Panics, while Democrats had 76 months of Depressions, Recessions or Panics. The highest peak unemployment was under President H. Hoover when peak unemployment reached 24.9 in 1933 during "The Great Depression," and the lowest was 1.9 Under F.D. Roosevelt in 1945. The shortest depression was under J.E. Carter lasting six months, and the longest was during the recovery from The Great Depression of five years two months partly under F.D. Roosevelt.

U.S. in Deficits-Recessions-Wars by U.S. Multi-Party

Year Actual-A Estimate-E	GDP- US $ billions	Federal Deficit $billions	U.S. Population	President	Wars	Recession
1960 A	543.3	4.79	179.323	J. F. KENNEDY		
1961 A	563.3	10.48	181.588		Bay Pigs War	
1962 A	605.1	7.15	183.881		Cuban Missile	
1963 A	638.6	4.76	186.204	L. B. JOHNSON		
1964 A	685.8	5.92	188.555			
1965 A	743.7	1.41	190.937		Dominican Rep.1	
1966 A	815	3.70	193.348		Dominican Rep 2	
1967 A	861.7	8.64	195.790			
1968 A	942.5	25.16	198.263			
1969 A	1019.9	-3.24	200.766	R. M. NIXON		2/1/69
1970 A	1075.9	2.84	203.302			
1971 A	1167.8	23.03	205.515			
1972 A	1282.4	23.37	207.752			
1973 A	1428.5	14.91	210.013			11/1/73
1974 A	1548.8	6.13	212.299	G. R. Ford		
1975 A	1688.9	53.24	214.609			
1976 A	1877.6	73.73	216.945			
1977 A	2086	53.66	219.307	J. E. CARTER		
1978 A	2356.6	59.19	221.694			
1979 A	2632.1	40.73	224.107			
1980 A	2862.5	73.83	226.546			1/1/80
1981 A	3211	78.97	228.670	R. REAGAN	Gulf Sidra	1/1/80
1982 A	3345	127.98	230.815			
1983 A	3638.1	207.80	232.979		Grenada	
1984 A	4040.7	185.37	235.164			
1985 A	4346.7	212.31	237.369			
1986 A	4590.2	221.23	239.595			
1987 A	4870.2	149.73	241.842			
1988 A	5252.6	155.18	244.110			
1989 A	5657.7	152.64	246.399	G. H. W. BUSH	Panama & 90	
1990 A	5979.6	221.03	248.710		Persian Gulf &-91	7/1/90
1991 A	6174	269.24	251.802			

Year	GDP-US $ billion 1	Federal Deficit $billions	U.S. Population	President	War	Recession
1992 A	6539.3	290.32	254.933		Somali Civil &94	
1993 A	6878.7	255.06	258.103	W. J. CLINTON	Bosnian War &95	
1994 A	7308.8	203.18	261.312		Haiti &95	
1995 A	7664.1	163.95	264.561			
1996 A	8100.2	107.43	267.850			
1997 A	8608.5	21.89	271.180			
1998 A	9089.2	-69.27 *	274.552	* Positive Deficit	Kosovo &99	
1999 A	9660.6	-125.61	277.966			
2000 A	10284.8	-236.24	281.422			
2001 A	10621.8	-128.23	284.184	G. W. BUSH	Afghan / Iraq &17	
2002 A	10977.5	157.75	286.974			
2003 A	11510.7	377.59	289.790			
2004 A	12274.9	412.73	292.635			
2005 A	13093.7	318.35	295.507			
2006 A	13855.9	248.18	298.145			
2007 A	14477.6	160.71	300.807		Great Depression	12/7/07
2008 A	14718.6*	458.55	303.492			12/8/08
2009 A	14418.7	1412.69"	306.202	B. H. OBAMA	Political Gridlock	
2010 A	14964.4	1294.37	309.348			
2012 A	16155.3	1086.95	313.998			
2013 A	16691.5	679.55	316.205			
2014 A	17393.1	484.60	318.563		ISIL/ Iraq / Syria &17	
2015 A	18036.6	438.49	320.897			
2016 A	18569.1	584.65	323.128			
2017 E	19161.9	602.51	325.374	D. J. TRUMP	Partisan Extremism	
2018 E	20013.7	440.16	327.636			
2019 E	20947.3	525.90	329.914			
2020 E	21980.6	487.95	332.207			
2021 E	23092.7	455.80	334.517			

U.S. wars from 1910 to 1959 are not included in this chart, which involved the Border War from 1910 to 1919; World War I from 1917 to 1918; the Russian Civil War from 1917 to1922; World War II from 1941 to 1945; Korean War from 1950 to 1953; and the 1953 Vietnam War. The above chart only shows wars from

1960 to 2017. There were twenty-two U.S. wars over eighty-five years during the twentieth and twenty-first-centuries.

The national debt of the United States is the amount <u>owed (Deficit) by the federal government of the United States</u>. The measure of the public debt is the value of the outstanding Treasury securities issued by the Treasury and other federal government agencies.

The <u>Gross Domestic Product (GDP)</u> in the United States was worth 18,036.65 billion US dollars in 2015. The GDP value of the United States represents 29.09 percent of the world economy. GDP in the United States averaged 6,560.26 USD Billion from 1960 until 2015, reaching an all-time high of 18,036.65 USD Billion in 2015 and a record low of 543.30 USD Billion in 1960.

Woodrow Wilson, a Democrat, served as the 28th President from 1913 to 1921 under a democratic majority through three consecutive elections before a Republican majority took over. His terms involved the U.S. in the First World War from April 6, 1917, to November 11, 1918, followed by the usual postwar economic surge in the economy that preceded the *"Roaring Twenties."* Shortly after Warren G. Harding was elected to become the 29th Republican President from 1921 to 1923, with a Republican majority, he died from a heart attack — thereby appointing the Vice-President Calvin Coolidge President from 1923 to 1929. The Great Stock Market Crash of 1929 began on October 24, known as *"Black Thursday,"* followed by the Wall Street Crash that occurred on the following *"Black Tuesday,"* October 29, 1929. These two crashes occurred, eight-months after Herbert Hoover, a Republican, took the oath of office as President of the United States and he agreed to help the banks but refused to approve any government aid to the citizens, fearing it would promote socialism. What emerged was an uncaring President who'd let the citizens starve instead of releasing federal money to help the people. More than 9,000 banks were unregulated and uninsured when they were forced to close, taking with them more than $2.5 billion in U.S. citizen's deposits. *"Hooverville"* was the name given to the many *"Shantytowns"* constructed from scrap lumber and cardboard boxes during those early most difficult years of the depression. The overall jobless rate jumped to 25% in 1933 with another 25%, or two out of every four workers taking large wage

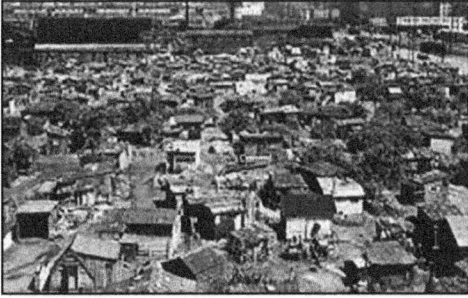

cuts or being asked to work part-time. Thousands of jobless workers lined up every day, for several city blocks, around almost every labor temple in every major city, hopelessly waiting to be chosen to obtain one of only a few part-term jobs. Many of these unemployed also stood in charity bread lines to feed their families until some ten years later when the start of World War II occurred on December 7, 1941. Some historians and economists blamed the increasingly uneven distribution of wealth and purchasing power as the cause of the *"Great Depression."* Congressman Louis McFadden, Chairman of the U.S. House Banking Committee and Currency Chairman (1920-31), said the following about the cause of the Great Depression:

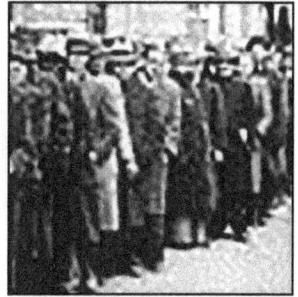

"It was not accidental. It was a carefully contrived occurrence...The international bankers sought to bring about a condition of despair here so that they might emerge as rulers of us all."

That included the new CFR. However, many citizens were just fed up with Hoover's *"hear nothing, see nothing, do nothing government."* In 1933, a Democratic presidential candidate from New York, Governor Franklin Delano Roosevelt promised change, saying: *"I pledge myself to a New Deal for the American people."* This New Deal used the power of the federal government to try and stop the economy's downward spiral, by waging war against the depression. Roosevelt shored up the banks by passing the *"Glass-Steagall Banking Bill,"* the *"Tennessee Valley Authority Act,"* the *"National Industrial Recovery Act"* and the *"Home Owners' Loan Act."* In Roosevelt's Inaugural Address and his *"fireside chats"* on the radio, his frequent contacts with the people helped to reshape their confidence. He said, *"The only thing we have to fear is fear itself."* Then in 1935, Roosevelt launched a second New Deal, which provided jobs for the unemployed by financing new public infrastructure projects like bridges, post offices, schools, highways, and parks. He also passed the *"National Labor Relations Wagner Act in1935,"* which gave workers the right to form unions and bargain collectively for higher wages and benefits. The *"1935 Social Security Act"* also helped the people purchase their own guaranteed pensions for older Americans and implemented unemployment insurance while providing federal help to care for dependent children and the disabled. In 1936, while campaigning for a second term, President Roosevelt told a roaring crowd at Madison Square Garden:

> *"The forces of organized money are unanimous in their hate for me – and I welcome their hatred ... I should like to have it said of my first Administration that in it the forces of selfishness and lust for power met their match, and I should like to have it said of my second Administration that in it these forces had met their master."*

In December 1936, the United Auto Workers started a forty-four-day sit-down strike at a GM plant that spread to over 150,000 auto workers in some 35 cities. By 1937, some 8 million workers had joined unions demanding worker's rights throughout the nation. By the end of the 1930's, the threat of the European war expanding to the U.S. loomed on the horizon and on December 7, 1941, the Japanese bombed Pearl Harbor causing the U.S. to declare war on Japan and then join its allies in what became World War II. Every physically capable man went to war, while *"Rosie the Riveter"* went to work to meet the new U.S. industrial war demands that helped to put an end to the Great Depression and the Dictator Adolph Hitler in Germany.

Since World War II, the U.S. financial problems have included the 1948 recession experienced by the shift to a wartime economy and the 1953 post-Korean War inflationary period. In 1957 the U.S. had to deal with a budget surplus of .08% of GDP and a 2.6% budget deficit. In 1959 the Federal Reserve raised interest rates, causing a minor recession before a slow but steady growth in the U.S. economy until 1969 when the U.S. finally started closing the deficits from the Vietnam War — causing the privately owned Federal Reserve to start raising interest rates. In 1973 the oil crisis caused the 1973-74 stock market crash, and rising unemployment — followed by an inflationary period in 1979 when the Iranian Revolution increased the oil price crisis throughout the entire world. In 1980, the peacetime expansion resulted in another inflationary period, causing the Fed's to again raise interest rates from 1986 to 1989, which lead to the 1990's becoming the longest period of growth in American history. However, the 9/11/01 terrorist attacks on the Trade Center brought this decade of growth to an abrupt halt. Then the subprime mortgage crisis led to the collapse of the housing bubble in 2009, leading to the Bear Stearns, Fannie May, Lehman Brothers, City Bank, and AIG 700 billion dollar bank bailout, which also required a 787 billion dollar government fiscal stimulus involving the GMC automobile bailout.

Back in 1810, the U.S. GDP debt ratio was 5%, and typical of wars increasing the debt ratio, the 1812 to 1816 war had increased the GDP debt ratio to a high of 15%, which did not return to 5% until 1830. The Multi-party politics at that time was failing, just as the U.S. is failing today, and that's when the Multi-party Congress previously became dysfunctional, forcing James Madison to reorganize the government into a single party that resulted in the *"Era of Good Feelings."* This new single party change successfully stopped the two-party partisan conflicts and maintained a debt ratio of 1 to 3% until 1850. Then partisan politics once again resurfaced between the Democratic and Republican members of Andrew Jackson's "Democratic" party and Henry Clay's "Whig" party. The debt ratio remained at 3% until the Civil War was started in 1862, causing a 15% GDP by the time the war ended in 1866. But after the Civil War, the GDP grew to 30% until 1870, when it returned to 11% until April 2nd, 1917 when the U.S. entered World War I — causing the GDP to reach a new high of just under 40% for the next ten years when it finally returned to 17%. Then when the 1929 Great Depression began, the GDP spiraled to 50% until just before the Japanese attacked Pearl Harbor on December 7th, 1941. Many of the citizens were still blaming both the depression and World War I on the wealthy faction's continued desire to gain greater control of the U.S. democracy since the wealthy faction first took over the Federal Reserve in 1913. On top of that, based on a Congressional Committee's report, General Smedley Butler on July 17, 1932, was approached by several wealthy representatives, asking him to help overthrow this nation's democracy in a military coup.

Then in 1946, after the end of World War II, the GDP debt ratio reached the highest ever at 114%, with a series of some twenty wars since then. The U.S. in 2017 is at 105%, with a Federal Debt of $20,533,379,940,805.47 — which is the gross outstanding debt issued by the United States Department of the Treasury. Many accountants are projecting the debt to reach an un-payable 40 trillion dollars in ten years, which suggests that the people will be left to pay for the resulting budget deficit. Today's Federal Debt per person is $62,928 which does not include state and local debt, or "agency debt" — nor does it include unfunded liabilities of entitlement programs like Social Security, Medicare, and Medicaid, Education, Infrastructure, or the current unfunded cost of this nation's defense. Yes, it is today's dysfunctional two-party system that has once again severely split the Republicans and the Democrats, as well as the people who love their democracy they are so close to losing. It is this same Multi-party and CFR destruction of our Democracy that has intentionally created this type of *"Authoritarian Fascist"* leadership the wealthy faction has been seeking since 1913.

Wars, Recessions and Partisan Extremism promoted by the many outside wealthy factions have provided Congressional political favors throughout the latter half of the twentieth-century, which is the major cause of this country's budgetary failure. These budgetary failures over the last three Presidential terms are now demanding proper annual business like budgeting, as well as more simple taxation to be accomplished if the U.S. ever intends to recover its Democracy. The Multi-party Congress defies all standards for treating budgeting and taxation the way a successful business would. In following normal government standards, a recent poll identified George Washington, Thomas Jefferson, Abraham Lincoln, Theodore Roosevelt, and Franklin D. Roosevelt as the top five Presidents, while it identified Herbert Hoover, George W. Bush, and Donald Trump as the worst leaders. Pulitzer Prize-winning Republican historian Jon Meacham predicted that the 150-year duopoly (Multi-party) Republican and Democratic control of Congress would soon have to end. And Joe Scarborough, a former member of the Republican Congress, who now hosts *"Morning Joe,"* on MSNBC said:

> *"Political historians will one day view Donald Trump as a historical anomaly. But the wreckage visited by this man will break the Republican Party into pieces — and lead to the election of independent thinkers no longer tethered to the tired*

dogmas of the polarized past. When that day mercifully arrives, the Multi-party duopoly that has strangled American politics for almost two centuries will finally come to an end. And Washington just may be able to work again."

On July 11, 2017, Scarborough announced on *"The Late Show"* with Stephen Colbert that he was leaving the Republican Party to become an Independent, supporting Independent policies.

Under the current Multi-party leadership, the U.S. has experienced twenty-two wars, the destruction of almost all of the people's tax-supported entitlements and what little health care we have left, as the *"Far-right"* now threatens to repeal the people's privately owned *"Social Security."* If they accomplish this, they will usher this nation into a far greater depression than the 1929 Great Depression. More recently, this nation has also experienced the unbelievable invasion of a Russian Cyber Attack.

1 Congressman Louis McFadden, Chairman of the U.S. House Banking Committee and Currency Chairman (1920-31)

2 President Roosevelt speech at Madison Square Garden in 1936

3 Joe Scarborough, a former member of the Republican Congress, currently hosting "Morning Joe," on MSNBC

6

Taxation

After the Civil War, Congress passed the first American income tax in 1861 at a flat 3-percent on all incomes over $800.00. Later Congress modified this tax to a graduated tax that Congress repealed in 1872 by enacting a 2-percent tax on income over $4,000. However, this tax was struck down by the Supreme Court in 1894. Before the 1907 bank panic, the United States had no central bank, which resulted in Congress appointing an outside *"National Monetary Commission"* that included such potentates of international banking and corporation owners as J.P. Morgan, John D. Rockefeller, Paul Warburg, Otto Kahn, and Jacob Schiff. As a result, Senator Nelson Aldrich, who was the father-in-law of John D. Rockefeller, Jr., and Colonel Edward M. House engineered the establishment of the first privately owned *"Federal Reserve Banking System."* What's so shocking about this privately owned Federal Reserve banking system is its owned primarily by the Commission, which a majority of the working class does not understand — nor that the Federal Reserve is not subject to oversight by either the Congress or the President. Former incumbent William Howard Taft and numerous other members of the Congress had been vehemently opposed to any privately owned central bank or tax program. It's also very confusing that Article I, Section 8, of the U.S. Constitution, granted Congress the sole power to coin money and regulate its value.

On top of all this, the Commission also recommended this nation's current income tax by proposing *"the Central Bank Act of 1913."* This Act required a Constitutional Amendment by the Congress in that the national income tax had previously been declared unconstitutional by the Supreme Court in 1895. In any event, Congress reluctantly approved this income tax on only one percent of the income under $20,000, with the assurance that this tax agreement would never increase — which of course never happened. Today's totally out of control Multi-party *(Duopoly)* budgetary tax program has become so abusively managed by an unsupervised and dysfunctional Congress that it will take years to recover if the U.S. can survive financially that long. This proposed tax amendment was attached to a tariff bill on July 2, 1909, and was finally passed by Congress on February 25, 1913. Three-quarters of the states approved this amendment due to the generous exemptions and deductions, and less than one percent of the population paid income taxes at a rate of only one percent of net income. However, in spite of the promise to never increase the tax, the Multi-party Congress launched the current out of control and intentionally confusing tax system that citizens of the U.S. now unwillingly live with and do not understand. Many business managers believed this was intentionally done to confuse the citizens of this Democracy so the Congress could easily make tax increases in the future. Income and social security taxes currently make up 80% of the government's revenue, while the tax on corporate income accounts for 11%. The U.S. government got by without any outside financial advice for most of its previous history, without corporate tax until 1909, and no income tax until 1913 — or any social security tax until 1935. F.D. Roosevelt signed the Social Security Act on 8/14/35 during the depression, and the government collected and paid Social Security Taxes for the first time in January 1937, and then the regular ongoing monthly benefits started in January 1940. Social Security was originally just a retirement program for the primary worker under the 1935 law, and then in 1939 the law added survivor's benefits and benefits for the retiree's spouse and children, and in 1956 disability benefits were added. The original 1935 law also contained the first national *"Unemployment Compensation Program"* that aids the states for various healthcare and welfare programs, as well as the *"Aid to Dependent Children's Program."* Both the worker and the employer pay into Social Security as an *"employee benefits program"* and it would be irresponsible for the Congress to attempt to take over this valuable employee benefit the employees own by allowing profit insurance companies to add their profit to the current nonprofit cost-effective employee benefit plan. The Social Security Medicare entitlement benefit was passed on July 30, 1965, to offset the McCarran Ferguson Act, and beneficiaries first signed-up for this entitlement program on July 1, 1966.

The 11% income revenue from corporations is far less than required by trillions of dollars of offshore tax evasion the international corporations are avoiding to pay under the current international tax laws. The UN's *International Law Commission (ILC)"* should be pressured to stop this abuse through their 1994 appointed body of legal experts at the request of the UN's General Assembly, by representing the abused nations in the international criminal court.

Many feel it was no accident that World War One produced a huge national debt. World War I made large profits for Bernard Baruch, the head of the War Industries Board, and Cleveland Dodge, who sold munitions to the allies. The Rockefellers and Rothschild's and J.P. Morgan also loaned hundreds of millions of dollars to the U.S. to cover the resulting World War I debt that rapidly increased from $1 billion to $25 billion. Both Baruch and Rockefeller were reported to have earned more than $200 million in interest alone during the war, but more assuredly, Rockefeller had found a way to have his loans paid by this nation's tax dollars.

Keeping profit-seekers from profiting from the U.S. tax dollar was once a major goal of the U.S. government. The government felt an obligation to provide cost-effective human healthcare services and educational benefits to the people that pay 80% of the tax dollar. Then the Federal Reserve owners, (the CFR profit seekers), were allowed to invade the U.S. budget, like receiving payment for the many U.S. loans for the 22 twentieth-century wars that made these corporate and bank owners very wealthy. Although numerous Congress members strongly opposed the appointment of this 1913 wealthy Commission, their passive opposition failed and as a result, the profit seekers all hurried to seek more profits from the government. To pacify the Congress members that opposed this; it didn't take long for the profit-seekers lobbyists to provide kickbacks for those Congress members that worked for a salary to turn their head, regarding their Oath of Office. Today the U.S. has no Federal bank, and all banks in the U.S. are in a key position for the wealthy faction to loan money without being responsible for the U.S. budget.

*The federal government, and states and local municipalities all levy **income taxes** on personal and business revenue and interest income. In most cases, income* *tax brackets are progressive, meaning that the greater the income, the higher the rate of taxation. Today there is an unbelievable number of many different kinds of taxes, such as taxes on income, and taxes on property and goods and services. Shockingly Americans spend 29.2 percent of their income on federal, state and local corporate and individual income tax; property tax; Social Security tax; sales tax; excise tax; and so much more.*

Income Tax:

In 1935, the U.S. income tax form involved a one-page tax form consisting of 34 lines and two pages of instructions. Today's 1040 form has 79 lines and 211 pages of instructions. Instead of a single tax form, the IRS now has 199 tax forms. Taxpayers spent nearly 7 billion hours complying with the tax code in 2016, and nearly 90% of taxpayers need help filing their income tax, at the federal, state, and local levels.

At the federal level, the amount paid depends on one's income within one of the four marital categories shown in the following Federal Tax Chart:

2016 Individual Income Tax Rate Schedule

Tax Rate	Single	Married/Joint & Widow(er)	Married/Separate	Head of Household
10%	$1 to $9,275	$1 to $18,550	$1 to $9,275	$1 to $13,250
15%	$9,275 to $37,650	$18,550 to $75,300	$9,275 to $37,650	$13,250 to $50,400
25%	$37,650 to $91,150	$75,300 to $151,900	$37,650 to $75,950	$50,400 to $130,150
28%	$91,150 to $190,150	$151,900 to $231,450	$75,950 to $115,725	$130,150 to $210,800
33%	$190,150 to $413,350	$231,450 to$413,350	$115,725 to $206,675	$210,800 to $413,350
35%	$413,350 to $415,050	$413,350 to $466,950	$206,675 to $233,475	$413,350 to $441,000
39.6%	over $415,050	over $466,950	over $233,475	over $441,000

The **Federal Individual Income Tax Rate** has one of seven standard progressive tax percentages that range from 10% to 39.6% within each salary range for each marital category. Some states have no state tax while some charge state and or city tax, and there are credits one can earn called *"Earned Income Tax Credit (EITC)."* EITC gives a tax credit to low and moderate wage earners, but overall income tax has become progressively far more difficult over the last century.

Sales Taxes:

Sales Tax is a method for states and local government entities to raise additional revenue. Sales tax is the most equitable form of taxation because the tax is voluntary and it extracts more money from those who consume more. However, the poorer taxpayer believes they pay a larger percentage of their income in sales taxes than wealthier individuals do. Sales tax on goods and services purchased can vary by state. Clothing is taxed at one rate, while restaurant food at another — and staple commodities are often not taxable.

Excise Taxes:

Excise taxes on specific goods such as gas, cigarettes, beer, and liquor were designed to deter unhealthy behavior called "Sin Tax." The federal government excise tax charges 18.4 cents per gallon of gasoline and 24.4 cents per gallon of diesel fuel — and other *"Luxury Taxes"* are imposed on certain items, such as expensive cars or jewelry.

Payroll Taxes:

Both employees and employers have to pay Social Security and Medicare tax under the *"Federal Insurance Contributions Act (FICA)."* Under the Social Security tax, employees and employers both contributed 6.2% of one's wages, for a total employee benefits contribution of 12.4%. In 2013, the maximum earnings subject to the Social Security Tax was $117,000, and in 2011 and 2012, the amount employees had to contribute declined to 4.2% of wages for that two year period, which was to encourage people to spend more to improve the U.S. economy. Under the Medicare tax program, both the employees and employers are required to contribute 1.45% of wages for a total of 2.9% benefit from one's wages. Unlike Social Security, there is no maximum taxable wage, but workers who earned more than $200,000 had to contribute 0.9% more to the program. Self-employed individuals are liable for the entire 15.3 percent, although one-half of that can become a business deduction on a person's income tax return.

Capital Gains Tax:

The Capital Gains Tax is 20 percent on the profits made from a sale of an asset such as stock and bond transaction. Profits made from the sale of real estate are also subject to capital gains tax. Single homeowners may exclude up to $250,000 of a capital gain on the sale of a home that was one's principal residence for at least two of the five years before the sale — while jointly married couples can exclude up to $500,000.

Property Taxes:

Property taxes are based on the property's market value and can apply to automobiles, boats, recreational vehicles, airplanes, or other property, which are also deductible. Homeowners pay their real estate taxes either once a year or as a monthly fee with their mortgage payments.

Real Estate Taxes:

Real Estate Taxes are often subject to fluctuation based upon a jurisdiction's assessment of the worth or condition of the property, location, market value, based on the amounts allocated to the recipients of the tax. Real estate property taxes are only deductible if they are used to promote general public welfare, and cannot be used to improve or increase the property value. Homeowners can qualify for a mortgage interest deduction.

Estate Taxes:

Cash, real estate, securities, insurance, and business interests are considered part of a federal government's estate tax that is less than 40% for estates exceeding $5.34 million involving one's right to transfer property upon one's death. An Inheritance or Estate Tax at the state level depends on the relation to the deceased.

Gift Taxes:

All gifts of cash, company shares, or cars over $14,000 are taxable up to 40% when it involves transferring wealth between two living people.

User Fees:

User fees are assessed on a variety of services, including airline tickets, rental cars, toll roads, utilities, hotel rooms, licenses, financial transactions, and many more, depending on where one lives.

Corporate Income Tax:
A business can range from a sole-proprietorship, a general partnership, a limited partnership, or a limited liability partnership to a corporation. Corporations are an independent legal entity that is separate from the owners that control or manage them. Corporations are considered legal individuals under tax law, which involves business contracts and can initiate lawsuits or be prosecuted, and are required to pay taxes as a business entity. There are various types of corporate structures depending on the industry, the corporate goals, and the size of the staff involved, such as:

Sole Proprietorship:
A Sole Proprietorship has no incorporation forms to file or fees to pay to the government and avoids the double taxation that occurs in other forms of corporations. Paying Corporate earnings are made through the owner's income tax, and for estates exceeding $5.34 million, there is no corporate income tax. The owner is personally liable for everything done under the business' name, and the owner can be held liable for damages.

Partnership:
A partnership is where two or more individuals legally contract to do business together, and the income earned must be recorded on each partner's tax return. As with a sole proprietorship, the corporation pays no corporate income tax, but all partners are personally and legally liable for the actions of all general partners.

Limited Partnership:
In a Limited Partnership, all partners are liable for any partner's actions. A limited partnership has two types of partners that are called either general or limited partners. General partners are involved in the day to day operations of the company and share all liability of all the general partner's. Limited partners are "passive investors, angel investors, venture capitalists, friends, or family members." They contribute funds and are paid profits, but cannot participate in the management of the business.

Corporations and Limited Liability Corporations (LLC):
There are several types of corporations or limited liability business structures that can avoid some or all of the business liability undertaken in

a sole proprietorship or partnership. An LLC is a state business structure that mixes the benefits of sole proprietorships and corporations while removing some of the disadvantages. The owners of LLCs are members, and there can be any number of members, but there must be a managing member who is in charge of daily operations. Members are not personally responsible for legal judgments, but taxes pass through to their income taxes. Members are not required to have a board of directors or hold a shareholder's meeting every year.

Subchapter "C" Corporation:

Under a Subchapter "C" Corporation the owner and the shareholders buy stock and are taxed under the Internal Revenue Code, and the corporation can take tax deductions once as a corporate income tax — and again when the corporation pays the shareholder by salary, bonuses, or dividends. They can also write off the entire cost of benefits as a business expense, and these benefits are tax-free. The shareholder's liability is limited, and they do not stand personally liable for corporate debts or any charges for illegal corporate behavior. The shareholders elect a board of directors that make business decisions and oversee policies. In many states, the "C" corporation reports its financial operations to the state attorney general.

Subchapter "S" Corporation:

A Subchapter "S" Corporation is a legal entity where the income flows directly to the shareholder's income taxes, which is called "pass-through taxation," limiting the shareholder's liability to only one tax payment. The Subchapter S Corporation pays no corporate income tax on the profits of the company, and all profits and losses are passed on directly to the company's shareholders. The shareholders file individual tax returns and pay income tax on whatever share of profits they receive from the business. If the business has more than one shareholder, the business must file an informational tax return to provide details of the corporate income of each shareholder.

A *Corporate Tax*, or *Company Tax*, is a direct tax imposed by a jurisdiction on the income or capital of corporations or analogous legal entities. Many countries impose such taxes at the national level, as well as the state and the local level. The rate of corporate income tax paid by a business varies between countries, although since corporations are legal entities distinct from their owners and operators, have been taxed as if they were people. This tax is paid annually based on the corporation's tax accounting period, or fiscal year. In the United States, the corporate income tax rate is 35%, while the combined corporate tax rate is 38.92%. The United States taxes the profits of US resident corporations at graduated rates ranging from 15 to 35 percent. A Federal Alternative Minimum Tax of 20% charged on regular corporate taxable income with adjustments.

The *"Organization for Economic Co-operation and Development (OECD)"* lists the U.S. as the highest Corporate Income Tax Rate in the entire industrialized world that works together with 34 government democracies, and more than 70 non-member economies to promote economic growth and prosperity as well as sustainable development.

Corporate Income Tax for Organization for Economic Co-operation & Development

2013	
Country	Corporate Income Tax %
Ireland	12.5%
Slovenia	17.0%
Poland	19.0%
Hungary	19.0%
Czech Republic	19.0%
Turkey	20.0%
Iceland	20.0%
Chili	20.0%

2013	
Country	**Corporate Income Tax %**
Estonia	21.0%
Switzerland	21.1%
Sweden	22.0%
The United Kingdom	23.0%
Slovak Republic	23.0%
Korea	24.2%
Finland	24.5%
The Netherlands	25.0%
Israel	25.0%
Denmark	25.0%
Austria	25.0%
Greece	26.0%
Canada	26.1%
Italy	27.5%
Norway	28.0%
New Zealand	28.0%
Luxembourg	29.2%
Spain	30.0%
Mexico	30.0%
Australia	30.0%
Germany	30.2%
Portugal	31.5%
Belgium	34.0%
France	34.4%
Japan	37.0%
United States	39.1%

The state corporate tax runs between 0% to 12%, as shown here:
Some cities also charge tax ranging up to 9%.

2013	
State	**Corporate Tax %**
Alabama	6.5%
Alaska	9.4%
Arizona	4.9%
Arkansas	6.5%
California	8.84%
Colorado	4.63%
Connecticut	9%
Delaware	8.7%
Florida	5.5%
Georgia	6%
Hawaii	7.4%
Idaho	9.4%
Illinois	7.75%
Indiana	6.25%

In analyzing federal corporate income tax, and state corporate income tax, the many foreign trade tax issues, and the unbelievable number of all the other tax programs — the U.S. taxation programs are not only confusing but totally out of control. Such lack of control is because of the lack of leadership by the dysfunctional Multi-party Congress that intentionally keeps the citizens of this once great democracy confused. Such confusion permitted the dysfunctional and overstaffed Congress to hide their lack of supervision and management that is caused by the ridiculous U.S. budget. Yes, the U.S. Congress has failed to prepare or follow basic annual budgetary standards or follow a more efficient and sensible overall single tax appropriations plan, which requires this nation's Congress to provide adequate supervision and maintenance of a far more simple and efficient budget and tax system. This disastrous situation this country's Congress has created suggests we can no longer allow partisan politics to remain unsupervised by the people of each state. Income and expense must be balanced annually, and today's huge deficits must be immediately dealt with and brought to a reasonable level by a state-supervised Congress.

7

Foreign Trade

A long-term goal for the U.S and the many deprived countries of the world is to balance foreign trade and replace U.S. foreign aid through self-sustaining trade tax independence. Trade taxation has perhaps had somewhat of a beneficial effect on nurturing and developing the accountability of governments, but it is long overdue that all Democracies now be brought together to cooperate on trade tax policy, standards, rules, and regulations as recommended in 1991. The current illegal and corrupt solutions that control the flow of money in and out of international corporate *"Tax-havens,"* only prevents the development of a more comprehensive overall cost-efficient plan. Bermuda, the Cayman Islands, and many other tax-free locations have financially benefited substantially through their many illicit *"Tax-havens,"* and hopefully these nations can be forced to universally take back control under some form of an ethical international trade type tax program. The reason this has become such an enormous problem for the U.S. is the unprecedented rise in wealth and control by the top one percent of worldwide income earners, while the working class pays the U.S. trade tax deficits. It's hard to believe that these entrepreneurs hold so much money where it is unusable, which could help cure cancer, provide healthcare, and maintain the people's benefits if taxation was properly implemented to benefit the middle class in a country that professes equality. Senator Bernie Sanders stated during a speech at Westminster College on September 21, 2017:

> *"There is no moral or economic justification for the six wealthiest people in the world having as much wealth as the bottom half of the world's population, 3.7 billion people."*

These wealthiest six people own $462.6 billion and the bottom 50 percent own $409 billion, based on the Forbes billionaires list and the Oxfam January 2017 report.

THE SIX WEALTHIEST BILLION

Bill Gates	85.6
Jeff Bezos	80.8
Amancio Ortega	79.8
Warren Buffett	79.6
Mark Zuckerberg	69.4
Carlos Slim Helu	68.4
TOTAL	**462.6**

By paying off this country's Congress or some off-shore *"Tax-haven,"* this elite one percent of U.S. wealth and international corporations escape their tax responsibility. These tax havens are estimated to be holding more than eleven trillion unused dollars in the hidden offshore asset. These assets go untaxed and result in an annual loss of U.S. tax revenue estimated at 250 billion dollars. This annual loss could be fighting climate change; the world's catastrophic water shortage; this nation's decaying infrastructure; the energy crisis, the climate crisis. It could also help solve the world's exponentially growing population of seven billion human beings that is projected to grow to 26 billion by 2145 and the rapidly advancing poverty, which in the U.S. is estimated at 47 million people. These unused assets, which are secretly held offshore beyond the access to taxation, are equal to about a third of the world's total assets. The global annual cross-border loss of this illegal tax evasion has been estimated to be close to 1.6 trillion per year.

Worldwide democracies will need to universally band together and develop an interim method of financially eliminating these offshore *"Tax-havens"* by somehow replacing the current uncontrolled off-shore profits these countries receive, while the UN and the world economy restructures itself into an ethical and auditable corporate trade tax system. In any event, this continued theft of public assets must be brought to an end if the U.S. ever expects to regain its democracy and establish open and auditable transparency in the taxing trade arena involving all international corporations — so they will all equally pay their fair share of the tax burden. Is it any wonder why so many Congressional members become millionaires in less than five years from the benefits they receive from corporations and other wealthy factions that support this illegal tax evasion strategy?

Money Laundering:

Money laundering creates the appearance that large amounts of money obtained from illegal activities, such as drug trafficking or terrorist activity, originated from a legitimate source. These organizations are called, *"fronts."*

There are three steps involved in money laundering:

- *"Placement"* Is introducing "dirty money" into the financial system, through illegitimate or criminal means.
- *"Gymnastics"* introduces dirty money by way of a series of complex transactions called *"Layering,"* or *"bookkeeping,"* which attempts to conceal the source.
- *"Integration"* attempts to show that the acquiring of the money was in a supposedly legitimate manner.

The following are other common forms of money laundering:

Smurfing:

Where the individual or group involved breaks up a sizable amount of money and deposits the cash over an extended period in a financial institution, or smuggles a sizable amount of cash across borders to deposit this cash in offshore accounts where money laundering enforcement is not considered illegal.

Tax-Havens:

If taxes are high in one's country, the corporate faction can gain an advantage by registering a new shell corporation in another country. Many financial celebrities have also used this shell-like relocation to avoid paying income tax. A recent study determined more than $20 trillion hidden in some 85,000 offshore tax-havens.

Shell Companies:
Shell Companies are legally incorporated on paper, to funnel money through the shell company and avoid paying taxes even though the company provides no actual products or services. The company can buy or sell through this shell company and not report its international-involvement, which avoids paying taxes on any profits.

Equity Swaps:
Requires an official agreement between two individuals or companies to reduce their taxes by exchanging a gain or loss in assets without legally transferring ownership — *"LIBOR"* meaning short term, indicates the participants can expect a fixed return, either in one payment or at several predetermined payment points.

By Avoiding Tax on Capital Gains:
The sale of properties like shares automatically acts as a deterrent to investors paying capital gains tax by using the shares as collateral after purchasing options from an investment bank at a fixed rate. The capital gains tax avoided by this type of sale would take place with a cash transaction, thereby allowing them to repay the loan from the profits using the money or the shares.

Evading Estate Tax:
One way of dodging estate Tax is setting up a *"Grantor Retained Annuity Trust (GRAT),"* which is a trust fund, and any income earned over and above the interest is completely free of income and estate taxes.

Shell Trust Funds:
Subscribers to this type of "tax plan" pay money into a trust fund that accepts their money as *"donations."* The fund then offers its members cheap loans, which the borrowers never pay back. By disguising their salaries as loans, the members can write off much of their income tax, thereby allowing individuals to pay as little as 1% income tax per year.

Incorporating:
Because there are many advantages to being a company and fewer to being a wage earner, many individuals incorporate themselves to avoid

various forms of tax. By creating a corporation, one can pay themselves a small, interest-free wage, claim expenses, and reduce income tax.

Payments in Kind:
Payments-in-kind is now obsolete due to tighter regulations, which allows one valuable and tradable commodities, such as gold, or other consumer goods and benefits. These commodities can then be "sold" or "traded on" for additional commodities. Another method gives companies the option of paying investors in additional securities rather than cash.

Life-Insurance Borrowing:
Involves an individual taking out a policy with a large cash dividend, giving the individual involved a lot of leverage when it comes to borrowing. Many banks will lend up to 90% of the surrender value of the policy, and since this isn't income, it isn't eligible for income tax or capital gains tax.

Real Estate Borrowing:
By listing mortgages on one's property list allows one to borrow money against the value of those properties tax-free until the rental income equals the expenses. On a property valued at $1 million, one can borrow 75% of the equity, or $0.75 million of tax-free borrowing because it isn't income but a loan.

1 Senator Bernie Sanders' speech at Westminster College on September 21, 2017

2 Forbes billionaires list, the Oxfam report-January 2017.

8

Working Class Benefits

After reaching the largest budget breaking period in this nation's history, this country's working class is beginning to wonder if they'll ever be able to protect their *"Human Service Entitlements"* which their elected Representatives are trying so hard to take away. Many of these people appointed politicians are trying to force the average American's tax-related *"benefits"* into the open competitive market so they can individually receive benefits from the profits they create. Worse yet, if the working class is ever going to be able to protect their *"earned benefits,"* it will require knowledgeable and just leadership that is capable of differentiating between an *"Open Market"* and the once protected *"Noncompetitive Market"* — which is essential in maintaining a healthy and productive workforce. By moving the working classes' human services into the open market, these wealthy factions, the international corporations, profit health insurance, the pharmaceutical industry, and the dysfunctional U.S. Congress are allowing all these factions to steal directly from the public treasury — challenging the citizen's equality rights in their democracy. Allowing Congress to pass the McCarran Ferguson Act of 1945 was the first challenge that sought to profit from this nation's health care nonprofit entitlement benefit, and as we have now experienced, profit insurance has spiraled healthcare cost to an unbelievable level that is continuing to climb higher every year. This Congressional decision has also catapulted this nation's healthcare system from number one in the world to 32nd. These same profit seekers now want to allow profit into this nation's long-standing non-profit *"Social Security Entitlement Benefit Program,"* which the worker and their employer pay for jointly. Shockingly, Congress loans huge sums of money from Social Security to only partially pay the Congresses' undefined and improperly authorized growing debts they continue to create. While all this is going on, Congress has secretly and selfishly acquired their private government healthcare, retirement, and other secret benefit programs. Isn't it strange that these plutocrats promote a Democracy in other countries, while the people are losing their freedoms in the United States? They propose standards and regulations for China when Congress can no longer maintain non-profit entitlement standards for the Social Security Retirement Benefits Program. Hasn't this wealthy aristocracy and the "Far-right's" insatiable appetite for profit from these human service benefits overshadowed the working classes freedom and equality forcing the working class back into the same bondage that President Hoover led the people into before the Great Depression. Perhaps this is why these closely knit international investment bankers (the CFR) and international corporations keep this nation in such a high state of fear and denial with all their unjust wars, confusing tax programs, lies, and the overall deceit they create. Yes, it's time this democracy protects its workforce salaries and healthcare, education, and the numerous forms of nonprofit infrastructure benefits, which has previously been the backbone of this great nation's democracy. These promised services should never be taken from the working citizens or be allowed to make such services and benefits fair game to the open market, where the working class can be financially hurt. Nor should employee benefits ever be referred to as *"socialized"* or *"big government"* programs when these benefits are the sole property of the working class that has earned and paid their tax for them. Social Security is not only a retirement savings plan, but a universal non-profit people benefit that helps to protect workers, retirees, and their families from life's unknowns. Social Security benefits have been helping support retirees in old-age, as well as those who become disabled, widowed or orphaned. Social Security has been highly successful for more than three-quarters of a century and isn't going broke as most plutocrats suggest. Social Security provides:

- Disability assistance 16%

- Widowed and Orphaned assistance 10%

- Old Age support and assistance 73%

All Congressional Members are currently required to pay into the Social

Security Entitlement Program but have elected not to participate in receiving any benefits — because they have created their own exclusive non-profit federal programs (CSRS & FERS). Could this be why they say Social Security is going bankrupt and why so many Congressmen are so anxious to see Social Security be placed under a profit-centered insurance program so they can receive kickbacks? Social Security is not going bankrupt, nor is bankruptcy even possible. Because of the Congresses lack of annual budgetary adjustments, it could mean Social Security won't be able to meet all its financial obligations in two decades from now, but the plan is not going bankrupt. It currently is collecting more than it pays out, while its trust fund provides huge loans to the government that pays less than adequate interest. Due to potential demographic and economic changes, Social Security expense will begin to exceed income in the year 2021, and around the year 2033, the fund will be in trouble if *"no adjustments"* are made. But even then, the revenue Social Security collects each year would still be enough to pay out at least three-quarters of its current and scheduled benefits well beyond the year 2090. For Social Security to go bankrupt, one would have to ignore Social Security's revenue completely, and most profit-oriented companies would go bankrupt in only a few years if they ignored revenue and sat back and watched their expenses drive their assets down to nothing. That's the same mistake politicians have openly made when they suggest they also want to adjust this country's budgetary expense downward without considering this country's annual income adjustments. That's why all successful businesses routinely adjust their budgeted income and expense every year before the fiscal year begins. If one would look at the Social Security budget properly, they'd recognize they'd only have to adjust income for Social Security by 0.9% of GDP to make Social Security's revenues match up with its expenses for the next 75 years. Under normal budgeting, one would raise the overall Social Security rate, which current national polls support, and there are several other simple solutions. However, Congress wants to transfer this remarkably successful program to a profit insurance company so they can receive kickbacks from the profits they add to the cost of the program. And although many think Social Security adds to the nation's deficit, it does not, since it has its taxing source (Social Security Payroll Taxes) and cannot spend more than it earns.

9

The Federal Reserve Act

Before the 1907 Bankers' Panic *(Knickerbockers Crisis)*, the U.S. had no central bank until the wealthy faction created a *"National Monetary Commission."* As previously discussed, under the leadership of Senator Nelson Aldrich, who was the father-in-law of John D. Rockefeller, Jr. This Commission included J.P. Morgan, John D. Rockefeller, Paul Warburg, Otto Kahn, and Jacob Schiff, who recommended in 1913, the creation of a Central Bank and the establishment of a privately owned Federal Reserve System, which would not be subject to oversight by either the Congress or the President. The Commission changed the responsibility for the Congress to create money even though *"Article I, Section 8, of the U.S. Constitution"*, had granted the Congress the *"sole"* right to coin and control the value of money in this country. The new owners of this controlling stock in this privately held Federal Reserve now include the following wealthy factions of the Rockefellers; Morgan; Carnegie; Rothschild; Lazard; Seiff; Loeb; and Sachs families. In addition to their stock, these international investment banks and corporations are today in a position to coin money and regulate its value, making their huge profits by lending the Federal Reserve fiat money (money without a gold standard) which these international investment banks created by the stroke of a pen. And since these banks establish their policies, the government has inadvertently relinquished their tax dollars and their interest income to all these privately held Federal and Commercial bank owners. It's also important to note, the Federal Reserve pays the Bureau of Engraving and Printing approximately $23 for every 1,000 notes printed. One million dollars in fiat money cost the Federal Reserve $230 for which this New World Order then secures a pledge of collateral equal to the face value from the U.S. government. This collateral is the people's land, the people's labor, and the people's assets, collected by the people's *"Internal Revenue Service (IRS)."* By authorizing these private international banks to regulate and create money, recessions, depressions, and inflation — Congress has unwisely granted the power to create profits for them as well.

During the Great Depression, Franklin Delano Roosevelt was forced to take this country off the gold standard due to the depression, and without a gold standard there is no way to protect the people's bank savings should any inflation reoccur, so the dollar is regulated by the market this New World Order creates. Gold had previously served as one's protector of property rights, but today's out of control deficit spending has essentially opened the door to this NWO's marketing scheme of confiscating the majority of wealth — which today's wealthy factions have now gained control over.

Before Woodrow Wilson's appointment as President in 1913, he'd been persuaded to support this proposed Federal Reserve Act and this country's first income tax, which he later admitted was a mistake. In 1885 the Supreme Court had declared that any form of a national income tax was unconstitutional, so this tax amendment required a constitutional amendment, which secretly, or illegally passed in Congress based on the efforts of Senator Nelson Aldrich. However, as presented to the American people, it seemed reasonable to create a small income tax on only one percent of income under $20,000, with the assurance that it would never increase — which never happened. What happened was John D. Rockefeller had assured himself that his Government loans were paid, which started this corrupt scam of profiting from the government's tax dollars.

In 1932, it's important to remind you a total overthrow of the Government was attempted, much like we see today when a group of this country's wealthy factions and corporations attempted to unseat President Roosevelt in a plot publicly exposed by retired Marine Corps Major General Smedley Butler at the McCormack-Dickstein Congressional Committee meeting. In his testimony, he told this committee on July 17, 1932; several wealthy men approached him who had asked him to help overthrow this nation's democracy in a military coup. In the Congressional

Committee's report, it validated Butler's allegations, but no prosecutions or further investigations ever followed — which is always what happens when it involves this upper crust. In retrospect, the devastation of the Great Depression had caused many of these very powerful and wealthy factions and international corporations to question the foundation of a Democracy — considering Fascism, Socialism, or even Communism as an alternative that would give them greater control over their wealth. They also achieved substantial control over much of this nation's gold since the U.S. had gone off the gold standard. Today, this power faction continues to aggressively seek total control over the *"World Market,"* the *"International Industrial Complex,"* and this nation's *"Armed Services."* And although the U.S. has the most powerful armed services in the world, the people are constantly being told the U.S. has to maintain this most powerful and expensive armed service in the world — when both the Congress and the Administration have admitted that terrorism can no longer use conventional weapons. With all this budget-breaking spending, we find nothing meaningful being done to adequately protect our troops, our borders, our port authorities, or even the implementation of our *"Homeland Security Report"* — for which the U.S. has received a second failing grade. From 2000 to 2008 the neo-conservatives took us into an unjust war with Iraq, which also took us from a $236 billion surplus to a $13.62 trillion debt. This debt is held by the people, while Intra-governmental holdings were at $5.34 trillion, for a combined total gross national debt of $21.97 trillion as of December 31, 2018, which is largely due to the high interest rate Americans pay the Federal Reserve. Worse yet, this huge debt is expected to increase some ten trillion dollars over the next ten years under the current Republican administration, and yet our Congress does nothing! So just where has all this bank loan and interest money gone that continues to add to the U.S. debt at a rate of more than two billion dollars a day? One also has to ask just why our dysfunctional Congress votes to rebuild other countries when far too many American paychecks are decreasing as favored executive benefits and international corporate profits are soaring to unheard of new levels. This country's workforce is paying for all this while our representatives in Washington D.C. suggest the people reduce their entitlement benefits while being forced into lesser paying jobs as international corporations hire cut-rate foreign help. The real question that needs to be solved is, doesn't this type of debt assure the eventual failure of having any benefits for the people in their future, thereby creating a communist type nation?

A trade deficit is when a country imports more than it exports, creating a negative balance of trade, which compares a country's exporting of goods and services with its imports. A trade surplus is when exports are greater than imports. To calculate the trade deficit, one must subtract the total value of exports from the total value of imports. The U.S. trade deficits started to grow disproportionately as early as 2000, going from $409 billion to $705 billion in the 2008 depression. Since then, trade deficits have been growing from $400 billion in 2009 to $502 billion in 2016. The following shows the trade deficit under the last three Presidents from 1996 to 2016:

Clinton Presidency: 1996 $184 billion – 1997 $198 billion – 1998 $298 billion – 1999 $372 billion

Bush Presidency: 2000 $409 billion -2007 $830 billion – 2008 — $705 billion

Obama Presidency: 2009 $383 billion – 2010 $494 billion – 2011 $548 billion – 2012 $536 billion – 2013 $461 billion – 2014 $410 billion – 2015 $500 billion – 2016 $502 billion

As most citizens already know, the United States has been running consistent trade deficits for more than thirty years, with no congressional attempt to reach a solution, even though Congress knew this country's high imports of oil and other consumer products were the cause. The largest trade deficits have been with China, Japan, Germany, Mexico and Saudi Arabia — while the United States has at times reached record surpluses with Hong Kong, Australia, Netherlands, and Belgium. These U.S. trade deficits coupled with the huge off-shore tax fraud that's benefiting so many international corporations are all occurring while the U.S. is obtaining high-risk loans from international bankers. These deficits and loans are seriously degrading the U.S due to the following ineptly defined and administered agreements that need far greater definition if the U.S. ever hopes to stop the damage they are causing to this nation's public treasury:

- The General Agreement on Tariffs and Trade (GATT - 1947)
- The North American Free Trade Agreement (NAFTA – 1994)
- The World Trade Organization (WTO- 1995)
- The Free Trade Areas of the Americas (FTAA - 1998)
- The Central America Free Trade Agreement (CAFTA - 2017)

On top of all this, many U.S. international corporations are continuing to export jobs from America — while this enemy within intentionally and uncontrollably reduces salaries that once favored the people. It's hard to believe that these privately owned aristocracies and the recent foreign cyber-attacks are all occurring under this sovereign nation's *"International Monetary Fund"* that is under control of the wealthy faction's privately held *"Federal Reserve"* and their many *"World Banks.* The U.S. is on a path toward a *"Dictatorship"* involving a variety of ideologues like the *"Republican Alternative Right, (Alt-Right)"* that favors the wealthy, the international companies, and countries like Russia that seek to flatten the United States. Therefore the U.S. has become easy prey for those Fascist countries that are standing in the wings waiting to see this once great nation fail. Isn't this playing directly into the *"enemy-within hands?"* And all this is occurring right out in the open, under every citizen's nose, while the wealthy leaders are intentionally maintaining a high level of terror and fear for a majority of the less secure U.S. citizens. Didn't the Napoleonic era in France, Caesar's Roman Empire, Spain, England, and the Hitler Regime all previously use this very same tactic? Ridiculous emotion filled phrases like the *"Rocket Man's Weapons of Mass Destruction"* or Vladimir Putin's complex Cyber-attack on October 7th, 2016 all expose their intent previously. Most of the nation's problems are almost always placed on the shelf until we legally study things further — which can go on for months and months because the enemy within completely controls this nation's leaders. Terror alerts are carefully designed to disorient this country while this nation's appointed leaders are doing nothing to protect the U.S. — when it's obvious the U.S. has more than enough hard evidence to stop this *"Enemy Within."* Haven't the people noticed that anyone that speaks out against such terrorism becomes a conspirator? Such military science may perhaps blind some of the population for a period, but there must be a growing and dissenting population that's not blinded by such tactics.

In studying this nation's long-term financial dilemma, we should also look back to 2015 when the *"International Industrial Complex"* with all their wealthy and crooked CEO's got into trouble because of their reckless corporate deregulation, which is now spiraling costs totally out of control. Where has the *"Justice Department,"* the *"Security Exchange Commission (SEC),"* the *"National Association of Securities Dealers (NASD)"* and this country's dysfunctional Multi-party Congress been regarding this deregulation of corporate ethics and standards? Isn't this the same as the scandal in 2015 that exposed hundreds of corporate crimes known as *"The Great Cover-Up?"* Worse yet, Americans saw only minimal evidence of any justice for those CEO's who severely damaged the working class by their many illegal acts. Why is nothing being done again, as the enemy within intentionally stalls all legal action against what is obvious corruption? Almost all this rampant corporate deregulation that today's President is proposing has already stimulated far too many ruthless international corporate executives into a false type of financial self-adoration.

10

Debt and Expenditures

The *"General Accounting Office (GAO)"* is the audit, evaluation, and investigative arm of the United States Congress legislative branch of the Government under the (*"Budget and Accounting Act of 1921"*). The GAO is to investigate all matters relating to the receipt, disbursement, and application of public funds. This office prepares reports to both the President and Congress and makes recommendations for the economy or efficiency involving all public expenditures, thereby attempting to help Congress meet its constitutional responsibilities to improve the performance and accountability of the federal government for the benefit of the American people. The GAO conducts financial and performance audits and sets standards for audits of government organizations, programs, activities, and functions while serving as the taxpayers' congressional watchdog to expose government waste and inefficiency. They also review government assistance received by contractors, nonprofit organizations, and nongovernmental organizations. The *"Comptroller General"* is appointed for a 15-year non-renewable term to head the GAO by the President based on the advice and consent of the Senate. To date, there have been only seven Comptroller Generals, and the President is unable to remove this official from office. However, this position may be impeached or removed by a joint resolution by Congress. The GAO standards are called the *"Generally Accepted Government Auditing Standards (GAGAS)"* and are followed by all auditors and audit organizations as required by law, regulation, agreement, contract, or policy.

The following GAO reports are available at (www.gao.gov), except those selected reports that protect national security and whose distribution is limited to official use only:

- *Federal Budget/Fiscal Issues to Financial Management*
- *Federal Education/ Retirement Issues*
- *Defense*
- *Homeland Security*
- *Administration of Justice*
- *Health Care*
- *Information Management and Technology*
- *Natural Resources*
- *Environment*
- *International Affairs*
- *Trade*
- *Financial Markets*
- *Housing*
- *Government Management and Human Capital*

Each year the GAO issues an audit report on the *"Financial Status of the United States Government"* outlining its public debt. They also prepare a *"Federal Fiscal Outlook Report"* describing the deficit in a cash report rather than an accrual basis, which sets out four goals:

- *Current and Emerging Challenges to the Well-being and Financial Security of the American People*

- *Changing Security Threats and the Challenges of Global Interdependence*

- *Transformation of the Federal Government to Address National Challenges*

- *Maximization of the Value of the GAO*

It's already clear that at one year in their term the Majority Republican Congress currently favors the very wealthy .01% of the 400 richest Americans who now have more wealth than the bottom 61 percent of the population. So at one year, the U.S. Treasury manages the day to day U.S. Federal Debt through its *"Bureau of the Public Debt"* under two main categories:

- *Intra-governmental holdings that currently total $5.554 trillion owed to nearly 230 other federal agencies.*

Note: There are close to 230 Federal agencies that buy U.S. Treasuries - as of December 31, 2016 - the U.S. Treasury listed the following major holders of debt:

- *Social Security - $2.801 trillion-(and yet they tell us SS is going broke)*
- *Office of Personnel Management Retirement - $888 billion*
- *Military Retirement Fund - $670 billion*
- *Medicare —Federal hospital & Supplementary Medical Insurance Trust Funds-$294 billion*
- *All other retirement funds $304 billion*
- *Cash on hand to fund federal operations $580 billion*

- *Debt Held by the Public that totals $14,403 trillion.*

Note: Debt held by the Public — The following public groups buy U.S. Treasuries, bills, notes, bonds, Treasury inflation-protected securities (TIPS), Savings Bonds, and State and Local Government Series Securities

Organizations Purchase Amount
- *Foreign $6.004 trillion*
- *Federal Reserve $2,463 trillion*
- *Mutual Funds $1,671 billion*
- *State and Local Government &Pension Funds $905 billion*
- *Private Pension Funds $553 billion*
- *Banks $663 billion*
- *Insurance Companies $347 billion*
- *U.S. Savings Bonds $166 billion*
- *Other $1.662 trillion*

In that 30% of the U.S. Treasury debt is held in trust for the people's retirement in Social Security — if the U.S. were to default on the $5.554 trillion of intra-governmental holdings — the greatest harm would be to its own U.S. citizen, which the current dysfunctional Multi-party seems to favor placing at risk.

The Federal Reserve has no reason to own Treasury notes, but because of the many spiraling financial problems that started in 2007, the Fed's and G.W. Bush needed to stimulate the economy by buying Treasury Notes, which would help to keep the interest rates low and help dispel the seriousness of the 2008 recession. Because the Fed can create credit with fiat money out of thin air — if the U.S. ever expects to take the debt off the balance sheet, the U.S. needs to resurrect the *"Gold or Silver Standard"* soon and stop this ridiculous creation of fiat money by the Federal Reserve. According to the February 2006 U.S. Treasury report and Foreign Holdings of U.S. Treasury Securities as of December 17, 2012, and a report for foreign countries as of October 2012, the following foreign countries hold U.S. Treasury Securities (debt) as follows:

Country Debt

- *China*   *$1.146 trillion*
- *Japan*   *$1.091 trillion*
- *United Kingdoms*   *$640 billion*
- *Ireland*   *$302 billion*
- *Brazil*   *$270 billion*
- *The Cayman Islands* *$254 billion*
- *Luxembourg*   *$212 billion*
- *Belgium*   *$98 billion*

Note: Switzerland, Hong Kong, Taiwan, Saudi Arabia, and India which each hold $130 to $244 billion. Both Japan and China want to keep the value of the dollar higher than the value of their currency, which keeps exports affordable for the U.S., and which helps their economies grow.

History of U.S Gross Federal Debt

YEAR	TRILLIONS
2007	*$8.95*
2008	*$9.99*
2009	*$11.88*

2010	*$13.53*
2011	*$14.76*
2012	*$16.05*
2013	*$16.72*
2014	*$17.79*
2015	*$18.12*
2016	*$19.5*
2017	*$20.4 (estimated)*

Note: Gross Federal Debt: Is the gross amount of debt outstanding issued by the US Treasury. "Debt held by the public" and "debt held by federal government accounts" are components of Gross Federal Debt.

11

Contracts

Competition in U.S. federal procurement contracting has become a major concern because of the sizable increases and the alleged misconduct involving the selection of noncompetitive contracts, which has been going on for far too long. Officials within the *"Department of Defense (DOD)"* have supported a reduction in the growing number of noncompetitive contracts, yet nothing has been done to correct this very serious problem when the DOD involves some 70% of the annual federal government's procurement spending. The 1984 *"Competition in Contracting Act (CICA)"* was approved to oversee competition in federal procurement contracts. So any procurement contract not entered into through the use of proper procurement procedures that are supported by statute, are subject to oversight by the CICA.

Full and open competition through the use of competitive procedures is required unless certain circumstances exist that would permit agencies to use noncompetitive procedures. (whatever that means?) All contracts entered into without full and open competition are also considered noncompetitive, but the loophole is that noncompetitive contracts can still comply when circumstances are permitting other than full and open competition exists, such as:

- *There is only a single source of goods or services*

- *There is an unusual and compelling urgency*

- *It involves products safeguarding the industrial base*

- *It must meet requirements of international agreements*

- *It involves legislative consent or purchase of brand-name items for resale*

- *It involves national security*

- *It involves contracts needed in the public interest*

And so here again, there are far too many loopholes and the management is so decentralized it is almost impossible to provide adequate supervision or enforcement. Full and open competition usually involves the use of sealed bids that are considered competitive proposals, but loopholes are still far too prevalent in what has now become a political quagmire. And on top of all this, the CICA has far too many escape clauses that permit agencies to employ simplified product value procedures that confuse things even more, such as:

- *When acquiring goods or services whose value is less than $150,000, or commercial goods or services whose expected value is less than $6.5 million, which can be increased to $12 million in the case of an emergency, when the procurement can vary from standard procedure.*

Another confusion involves the issuance of orders under *"Task Order or Delivery Orders (TO/DO)"* not considered under CICA supervision, even though the awarding of a TO/DO contract is under CICA supervision. In 1994, the *"Federal Acquisition Streamlining Act (FASA)"* established a preference for multiple-award (TO/DO) contracts to include:

- *The requirement that agencies are to provide contractors a fair opportunity to compete for orders (under multiple-award contracts) more than $3,000.*

The *"Government Accountability Office (GAO)"* has also been authorized to:

- *Oversee orders that increase the scope, period, or maximum value of an underlying contract.*

93

And the *"National Defense Authorization Act (NDAA)"* for the fiscal year 2008 further limited the use of single-award (TO/DO) contracts that:

- *Specify what constitutes a fair opportunity to be considered for orders more than $5.5 million under multiple-award contracts and also granted GAO jurisdiction to hear protests of orders valued more than $10 million.*

Note:

The provision authorizing GAO to hear such protests regarding the orders of civilian agencies came to an end in May 2011. The 111th Congress enacted legislation extending the sunset date for GAO's jurisdiction over protests of orders valued more than $10 million issued by defense agencies until September 30, 2016 (P.L. 111-383, §825).

With all this Congressional chaos is it any wonder why we need to urgently take action to protect this nation's budget and stop the earmark kickbacks from the wealthy corporate factions.

Public officials and politicians also present a serious growing problem:

Richard Cheney served as Secretary of the DOD from 1989 to 1993. During his Vice-Presidency, which began on January 1, 2001, he was referred to as the "Eminence grise," for a good reason. Then from 1997 to 2001, while not in a government position, he served as the Chairman and CEO of the Dallas-based energy service company Halliburton, where it has been estimated he enriched his well-being by some forty-million dollars during his four years at Halliburton. While Cheney served as Vice-President, Halliburton was under investigation by the SEC for falsely reporting cost-overruns as revenues to the tune of $100 million, which had occurred during Cheney's watch when he served as Chairman and CEO at Halliburton — overseeing the implementation of this potentially serious accounting fraud that occurred in 1998. However, Cheney's more grievous and questionable example of potential conflict of interest related to the numerous non-competitive and open-ended bids that allowed $10.86 billion in tax dollars to flow to Halliburton while Cheney was serving as Vice- President. Here again, his involvement and the open investigation of potential abuse of awarding open-ended contracts to favored corporations have seen only a very few CEO's or plutocrats *ever go to jail. Senators and House Members that seek personal favors for themselves or their state are far too closely involved in this highly disputed bid process, and this type of abuse must also be openly faced up to and brought to an end.*

12

Earmarks

In 2008, George W. Bush anticipated the Republican Party would lose seats in both the House and the Senate and sought to tighten the strings on the anticipated Democratic Majority so they would not be able to hide preferential personal favors they entered into with their various power factions. In 2011, the proposed G.W. Bush *"Earmark Transparency Act"* was presented to the Senate by President Obama with proposed amendments to the *"Congressional Budget Act and Impoundment Control Act of 1974"* to significantly modify the role of Congress in the Federal budgetary process. The proposal asked to create standing budget committees in both the House and the Senate and to establish the *"Office of Management and Budget (OMB)"* and move the beginning of the fiscal year from July 1 to October 1. It also requested the Secretary of the Senate, the Senate Sergeant at Arms, and the Clerk of the House of Representatives to develop a free *"Public Searchable Website"* that specified certain identifying information relating to *every request by any Member of Congress* regarding any congressionally directed spending or *"Congressional Earmarks."* Earmarks involve any congressional directive that designates funds for a specific project. This website requires that every request for a congressional earmark from a Member of Congress is made available on the website within five days after its submission to a congressional committee. Investigations on federal spending had found that this executive order intended to constrain *"abusive earmarking"* and *"politically pressured spending"* — which was not being enforced and was becoming more susceptible to political influence. As a result, these watchdog groups were asking (OMB) to enforce such an executive order and make communications between members of Congress and government agencies available to the public in regards to all spending on earmarks. The executive order placed on the requesting Member of Congress the burden of providing the required information promptly and compliance with this Act to the Secretary of the Senate and the Clerk of the House also placed on the chair of each committee the burden of providing:

- *The amount approved by the committee*

- *The amount approved in the final legislation (if approved)*

- *The name of the federal department or agency through which the entity was to receive the funding*

The U.S. does not have a spending problem so much as it has a corrupt Congress and an outside wealthy faction relationship that promotes and supports an out of control earnings problem for the .01% of the wealthy corporate factions and their owners. It also has a serious lack of adequate and well-defined free trade policies, such as the Congresses' profit-seeking McCarran Ferguson Act of 1945 and the recent *"Halliburton"* fiasco. The current lack of adequate professional pharmaceutical healthcare standards for the sick and disabled has overwhelmed every family's day to day budget. As a result of this unbelievable chaos, members of the House and Senate are only partially prohibited from inserting undefined earmarks into legislative proposals. Congress members are increasingly using emails, phone calls, letters, and personal visits to pressure other Members of Congress to make the desired politically favored funding decisions that were supposed to enforce the earmark transparency rule that was to improve public communications between Congress and the agencies in charge of disbursing funds for special projects. This executive order also stated that executive agencies should not commit, obligate, or expend funds by earmarks included from any non-statutory source, including requests in reports of committees of the Congress or other congressional documents or communications from or on behalf of the Members of Congress. Such reports promoted the idea that all spending decisions should be made on their merits and in the sunshine, but what has happened is earmark decisions are now being made in secret, allowing political appointees and others to use federal monies to reward political allies and insider deal-making. The Congress needs to ensure that federal discretionary spending decisions are transparent and merit-based and enforce the *"Earmark Transparency Act"* that outlines a single searchable database of earmark requests to be submitted in writing and posted on the Internet under the *"Freedom-of-Information-Act."* Research has only confirmed that for years, federal agencies have been ignoring any binding type of executive order designed to protect taxpayer dollars from being misused.

It is this very same type of Congressional financial deregulation that had destroyed Clinton's annual budget surplus through the capitalist's desire to profit from all the non-profit benefits we once provided to the middle class. This deregulation of trade standards for corporations, the ridiculous and unfair Bush tax cuts for the wealthy one-tenth-percent, the internationally corrupted cyber invasion of this nation's ridiculous electoral college election system, as well as this nation's uncontrolled wars associated with the capitalist's profiteering — have all added to today's dilemma. And on top of all this, we are now allowing these capitalist factions to create state-controlled social systems that severely penalize the median wage earners, who are the backbone of this once great democracy. And this is all happening while the top .01% of wealth is openly taking huge profits that are higher than anything ever experienced during the entire history of this nation. Yes, the Multi-party Congress has opened the door to the robber baron's elite oligarchy of international investment banks, and the disorganized NWO has been silently gaining greater world power and control during the last half of the twentieth century's amazing but also out of industrial control advancements. And more recently, the U.S. citizens have unwillingly supported the *"Troubled Asset Relief Program (TARP)"* through the citizen's tax dollars, rather than let these mismanaged privately owned power structures feel the pain of their mismanaged and misuse of the people's tax dollars to craft their overwhelming profits.

As Milton Friedman in his book *"Capitalism and Freedom"* said:

> *"Only a crisis — actual or perceived — produces real change."*

American citizens are unknowingly rewarding today's dysfunctional Multi-party partisan politicians for pouring this nation's financial stimulus into an oligarchy of capitalist corruption, where one's tax payments are being seized and misused under the guise of some fallaciously created crisis.

This type of panic legislation is bad legislation and today's close *"Alt-right"* Republican relationship with the many wealthy corporate factions that have intentionally created these actual crises have destroyed the financial well-being of this country's middle class. Because of Clinton's $236 billion budget surplus in the year 2000, George W. Bush felt it was time to revise the United States tax-code by signing into law the following three Acts:

- The Economic Growth and Tax Relief Reconciliation Act (EGTRAA) of 2001.

- The Jobs and Growth Tax Relief Reconciliation Act (JGTRRA) of 2003.

- The Tax Relief, Unemployment Insurance Reauthorization, and Job Creation Act, signed into law in 2010.

These three Acts were incorrectly thought to have significantly reduced the tax rates for all U.S. taxpayers, but this was not the case in that these tax cuts had failed to encourage growth and they seriously increased the budget deficit by shifting the tax burden from the rich to the middle class. Worse yet, these three Acts had sunset provisions that were due to expire on December 31, 2012, which they extended for two years by the 2010 Tax Relief Act. The planned spending cuts under the Budget Control Act of 2011also came into play as a compromise to resolve the congressional dispute concerning the United States debt ceiling and the unjustified failure of the 111th Congress to pass a federal budget, which resulted in the *"United States January 2013 Fiscal Cliff Situation."* A series of previously enacted laws were to come into effect simultaneously, which would increase the average citizen's taxes while decreasing spending to help resolve the Bush created depression of 2008. Under the Budget Control Act of 2011, it was the budget sequestration that was to reduce discretionary spending while making broad cuts for some of the Federal Agencies and departments other than Social Security, Medicaid and the U.S. military pay and pensions. If Congress had jumped off this dangerous Fiscal Cliff, it would have significantly increased the average citizen's tax rates and decreased most government programs, which could have cut the operating deficit in half at the expense of the average working American. The *"American Taxpayer Relief Act of 2012 (ATRA)"* partly addressed the revenue side of the Fiscal Cliff by implementing smaller tax increases following the end of the three Bush tax cuts that had caused this country's deficit problems in the early 2000s, but it did not provide a solution. As a result, intense debate and media coverage of the Fiscal Cliff drew widespread public attention by the end of 2012 due to its destructive and unrealistic short-term fiscal and economic impact. With the passage of ATRA, the CBO projected a more realistic 8.13% increase in revenue and a 1.15% increase in spending for the fiscal year 2013. It also projected a $157 billion decline in the 2013 deficit, rather than the unrealistic sharp $487 billion decrease projected under the Fiscal Cliff proposal that would have seriously hurt the average working American. On January 1, 2013, the U.S. did go over the cliff, but on that same day, the Senate and the House were forced by common sense to pass compromise legislation that President Obama signed into law the following day. And as a result, the dysfunctional plutocrats in Washington were forced by public pressure to delay what could have been a disaster for the average American worker and the U.S. economy.

The Plutocrats in Congress have been bought off and no longer represent *"We the People."* The huge corporate campaign donations that have far exceeded even the most shameful level made more than half of this nation's Congress millionaires in less than five years for those that sought wealth over equality for all. Americans must get outside money out of politics. Yes, this nation's financial system is badly broken, based on an unsustainable U.S. dollar and the uncontrollable Federal Reserve's excessive creation of fiat money. And now that many of these politically appointed and unsupervised members of Congress have become corrupted, it will require the weeding out and incarceration of all the crooks that have benefited before we can eliminate this fraud created by this privately owned and controlled Federal Reserve and their overpaid politicians. Americans all know the answer is transparency, reform, and equal justice for all under this nation's rule of law — and although this may never take place, it must be attempted soon if we ever expect to take back this nation's democracy. The current President's authoritarian dictatorship and the Republican's Far-Right intend to repeat this 2000 to 2008 depression, all because the public has yet to find its voice.

1 Milton Friedman's book *"Capitalism and Freedom"*

13

Concerns That Matter

This Chapter outlines numerous obstacles to the U.S. remaining a democracy that protects the equality of *"We the People"* — and this freedom may soon perish if the people do not strongly resist what some 15,000 scientists from 184 countries published in November 2017 in the Journal of BioScience. William Ripple, an ecologist from Oregon State University, said:

"Soon it will be too late to shift course from our failing trajectory."

The Government's National Climate Assessment report blames humans for what is currently happening in climate change. The number of ocean dead zones has increased, and amphibians and fish and other mammals have declined by nearly 30 percent. The water shortage; the decaying infrastructure; the energy crisis; the world's exponentially growing population all are reaching disastrous levels. The number of the world's rapidly advancing poverty, the exporting of jobs, and the many vitally important personal facts are all ignored by the current Multi-party Congress.

Climate:
The earth's average surface temperature has risen by more than a half degree Celsius since 1992, largely because of the increased carbon dioxide emissions that have increased by 62 percent along with other dangerous emissions released into the atmosphere. Sixteen of the warmest years on record occurred since 2001 with 2016 being the warmest year on record, and eight of the 12 months of 2016 being the warmest months on record. The oceans have absorbed much of this increased heat since 1969, while

Greenland lost 36 to 60 cubic miles of ice per year between 2002 and 2006 and Antarctica lost about 36 cubic miles of ice between 2002 and 2005. Glaciers are also rapidly losing ice from the Alps, Andes, Alaska, Africa, and the Himalayas and the Rockies. Global sea level rose about 8 inches during the twentieth century, which is nearly double that of the nineteenth century and the Arctic sea ice is also declining rapidly over the last thirty years. The acidity of the ocean's surface waters has increased close to 30 percent due to the two billion tons of carbon dioxide being released into the atmosphere every year. As a result, air quality has become a global issue as gaseous pollutants pass from continent to continent. Emissions from human activities, wildfires, and wind-blown dust all affect air quality. This global issue has required a universal satellite monitoring system, ground networks, and well planned universal airborne sampling systems. Geostationary satellites that can monitor a single location so that the instruments can accurately collect the changing data are also required. The factors that affect air quality include surface emissions, atmospheric transport, all the chemical transformation interactions and how they're changing over time are all essential for the monitoring of air quality. Aircraft are also involved in monitoring the air between 1,000 to 25,000 feet with remote-sensing instruments that simulate satellite observations while scientists are collecting data from their ground-based air quality monitoring networks. Oceans cover about 71 percent of the planet and even tiny changes in this huge body of water can cause enormous effects on climate and weather like we are currently experiencing in the increased intensity and frequency of hurricanes, tornadoes, rain, and flooding, as well as forest fires. A new study finds lightning storms have become the main cause of massive forest and building fires in Alaska and northern Canada, with the storms migrating north as climates warm. Studying the oceans has helped scientists to forecast climates and understand the current massive band of warm ocean water called "*El Niño*," which moves from west to east across the equatorial Pacific Ocean. El Niño has built up substantially over the years, causing abnormal weather patterns all around the globe as well as the rainy and cooler weather in the southern United States. The reverse of the El Niño phenomenon, called "*La Niña*," is directly associated with the drought in the Southwest. Arctic winter warming events are also becoming more frequent and are longer-lasting than three decades ago. Research shows the southern Amazon rainforest triggers its rainy season and establishes the close connection between the rainforest ecosystem and climate while Arctic winter warming events have become more frequent. Blending standard jet fuel with biofuel reduces soot emissions from airplanes, and this may reduce contrails and their contribution to global warming. May 2017 was the second-warmest May in 137 years of modern record-keeping, and research has shown how cost and damage from these weather disasters and smoke are all expected to impact the atmosphere and climate much more than previously thought. The President's withdrawal from the Paris Climate Agreement has already destroyed the respect the U.S. previously earned from other nations. But worse yet, Congress has done nothing to help ease these problems.

Water Shortage:

By the year 2025, an estimated 1.8 billion people will be living in areas of water shortage, and the current water stressed earth is expected to be under *"extreme drought"* by the year 2050. Surprisingly, close to 800 million people are living without clean drinking water, while one-third of the current African population lacks adequate drinking water. California will require three times more groundwater than currently available, and China will soon lack safe drinking water for almost 1/3 of its population. Worldwide, some 2 billion people currently rely on underground well water.

The world's population has doubled since 1975, and the water use has quadrupled while the population is estimated to add one billion people over the next ten years. In addition to this, the global middle class is expected to increase from 1.8 to 4.9 billion by 2030, which will require a major increase in freshwater consumption. The *"UN's Food and Agriculture Organization"* indicates that one in every five developing countries will experience water shortages over the next thirty years. Agriculture is expected to require a trillion cubic meters of extra water over the next ten year period and the *"International Energy Agency"* estimates that global energy will need to increase its freshwater needs by 35% while manufacturing needs are estimated to increase by some 400% over the next thirty years. Today's vitally important thermoelectric power plants currently use almost 50% of all freshwater. The U.S. Ogallala Aquifer is the largest aquifer in Texas and the High Plains Region, which is being used at a rate far exceeding the water it replaced. The Colorado River Basin has lost almost 65 cubic kilometers of water over the last ten years.

There is already increasing transboundary conflicts over river water ownership. Currently, some 4.5 billion people throughout the world depend on some water source that is either currently becoming polluted or running dry. Humans require close to 12 gallons of water a day to sustain a single life, and the average American currently uses about 158 gallons a day. According to the *"U.S. Intelligence Community Assessment of Global Water Security,"* by 2030, humanity's annual global water requirements will exceed the current sustainable water supplies by 40%. Water tables are rapidly declining where more than half of the global population lives, and in less than 25 years there will not be enough fresh water in the world to meet the global population's needs if humans do not make the necessary changes. Worse yet, the Multi-party Congress has done nothing to help ease this problem or investigate the possibility of efficiently desalinizing sufficient salt water to help solve this dilemma.

Decaying Infrastructure:
America's infrastructure is in a state of crisis. Some roads, trains, and subways are over 100 years old and are perilously in need of repair and are currently costing the country billions of dollars in economic growth. Street potholes and tunnels are becoming increasingly dangerous. The sewage systems need proper maintenance, and replacement — and the electrical grids, gas, and oil pipelines need repair and maintenance. Ports, and freight transportation on roads and by rail, and internet broadband are all infrastructures that require constant attention. As a result, fixing the roads, bridges, tunnels, and transportation has now become a huge future cost item, not adequately provided for in the budget. The *"American Society of Civil Engineers (ASCE)"* inspects the conditions of the bridges, the water, and the transportation infrastructure every four years. In publishing its findings, the U.S. scored a D+ indicating that some 2,000 dams could break, some 56,000 bridges are in a total state of disrepair and are about to fall, and one out of every five roads needs repair. The director of the ASCE indicates that in three years, this nation will have lost over four trillion dollars of growth in GDP, and this aging infrastructure will cost each American family about $3,500 a year. Congress wants to privatize this repair and pay the added cost of profit to the wealthy, for what should be a government non-profit cost effective repair. Sound familiar? Just like we once asked Americans to pay what could have been private nonprofit health care tax-assisted non-profit health care. The

administration says they plan to spend trillions on infrastructure and yet the current budget allows for only $200 billion. Worse yet, the unsupervised Congress refuses even to discuss why the U.S. fails to include adequate maintenance in the U.S. budget and has here again failed this nation's infrastructure under their supervision.

Energy Crisis:

An energy crisis occurs when there is a significant reduction in the supply of energy throughout the world economy, such as electricity from the national electricity grids or the fuel required for vehicles. The global growth of the population and the industrial development has in recent years led to a huge increase in the world's demand for energy. The Middle East tension, the falling value of the U.S. dollar, the dwindling oil reserves coupled with the world's concerns over *"Peak Oil"* and oil price speculation — have all only added to the recent 2000 energy crisis. Over-consumption, trouble in the refineries, port tie-ups that restrict fuel supply, obsolete equipment, and ignoring all the significant weather changes will all reduce the fuel supply and have a substantial impact on price. *"Peak Oil"* has historically been the point in time when the maximum rate of petroleum extraction will occur, while *"Depletion"* refers to a period of falling reserves and supply after peak-oil occurs. After the peak-oil, oil is expected to decline steadily. *"World Energy Consumption"* involves the total yearly energy used for the entire civilization's across every industrial and technological sector in the world. World Energy Consumption will have deep implications for humanity's socioeconomic and political concerns. The International Energy Agency (IEA), the U.S. Energy Information Administration (EIA), and the European Environment Agency (EAE), all maintain and publish energy data on all the systemic trends and patterns in World Energy Consumption. These publications help to frame current energy issues and propose useful solutions to better avoid all the social and economic implications of the inevitable global decline in oil production.

The world needs to find alternatives before the peak oil crisis, and the greenhouse gas emissions occur — like developing an energy conservation plan or developing a fuel substitute. Another alternative would be to provide a fuel reserve like the *"United States' Strategic Petroleum Reserve,"* used in an emergency. Governments need to come to an international agreement regarding an orderly approach to this inevitable problem before it happens, thereby *"achieving the universal aspirations of humanity... based on shared principles and the rule of law."* For example, determining a series of oil and natural gas price hikes over the next two decades might help to reduce the overuse of oil. Additional nuclear power plants with liquid fluoride thorium reactors, and a type of *"Molten Salt Reactor"* could also replace the energy from peak oil, and the use of coal or gas should at least get a response from Congress now, not after the *Peak Oil* crisis finally rears its ugly head. Many other countries have already set deadlines for their transportation infrastructure to change to electric vehicles, and yet the U.S.'s dysfunctional Multi-party Congress fails to propose any policy for electric cars because they are protecting the auto manufacturers and the many gasoline industry benefits they currently receive.

Population Crisis:

The estimated U.S. population for 2016 was 322,762,018 according to the U.S. Census Bureau, meaning that the U.S. added more than 2.4 million people (0.77%) to the population in one year. From 2010, the U.S. population has increased by 14,016,480 or 4.54 percent. In 2015, the annual projected world population was 7,295,889,256, having increased by 1.08 percent (or 77,918,825). And today's seven billion human beings are projected to grow to 26 billion by 2145, while the total world population is growing faster than the U.S. Over one year, the U.S. is projected to birth one person every eight seconds, while the death of one person occurs every 10 seconds. Immigrants are adding a new person to the population every 29 seconds, so births, deaths, and international migration are increasing the U.S. population by one person every 17 seconds. However, the 2008 recession has had a drastic impact on U.S. birth rates, and recently, there are also fewer immigrants. Overall, fewer births and immigrants have brought down population projections substantially, according to the latest population projections from the Census Bureau. Couples have also been getting married later in life, and in 2011, the median age at first marriage was 28.7 for men and 26.5 for women, which is the highest age on record. As a result of this rising age factor, there is an increase in the number of women in their early 40s remaining childless, which the U.S. Congress is well aware of but as usual ignores. The U.S., like most other Western Nation-States, makes no adjustment to one's pension (Social Security) for retirement even when the older retirees outnumber the younger workers. Worse yet, this ignores all the items described in this chapter that will most likely have to be adjusted because we are knowingly depopulating the U.S. and not adjusting the projected budget or tax accordingly. Isn't it just a bit shocking that the U.S. Congress no longer considers it even necessary to adjust the budget or tax annually?

Poverty:
"Poverty" is the state of an individual who lacks a certain amount of material possessions or money based on social, economic, and political elements. *"Absolute Poverty"* refers to the lack of the means necessary to meet basic needs such as food, clothing, and shelter. *"Relative Poverty"* occurs when people do not enjoy a certain minimum level of living as compared to the rest of the population. Changes in poverty often relate to the industrial and agricultural ability to yield enough food or products to reduce their cost. In 2015 the U.S. poverty was estimated at 43.1 million people, and the poverty rate was 13.5 percent, as measured by U.S. Census Bureau. The poverty estimates do not include those who are homeless, and it also excludes military personnel who do not live with at least one civilian adult. While poverty fluctuates from year to year, so do incomes relative to the Federal Poverty Level (FPL). In 2015, 19.4 million people's household income was below 50 percent of their 2015 poverty threshold. These individuals represented an estimated 6.1 percent of all Americans and 44.6 percent of those in poverty. Poverty rates in the U.S. have ranged from a high of 22.4 percent in 1959 to a low of 11.1 percent in 1973, and these rates usually fluctuate somewhere between 11 and 15 percent. Fluctuations in and out of poverty also happen more often after life events such as a marriage, divorce, or a sudden change in income occurs, which closely correlates with unemployment and wage statistics.

The 1972 *Women, Infants, and Children (WIC)*, and the *U.S. Department of Health and Human Services (HHS)* updated their guidelines in 2017 — trying to develop their *Federal Poverty Guideline (FPG)* on income thresholds based on this nation's poverty measurements. Since the 1960s, new poverty measure includes the U.S. Census Bureau's measurement, which has provided a more complex understanding of poverty in the U.S. This supplemental measure includes basic costs of living that vary across states. It also considers transfers from safety net programs and in-kind benefits. The FPG is one of the income criteria that the *Low-Income Home*

Energy Assistance Program (LIHEAP) grantees can use in determining household eligibility. Grantees can establish the maximum household income for LIHEAP eligibility at either 150 percent of these federal poverty guidelines, or at 60 percent of *State Median Income (SMI)*.

Federal Poverty Guidelines for FFY 2017

Size of family unit	100% of Poverty	110% of Poverty	125% of Poverty	150% of Poverty	175% of Poverty	185% of Poverty	200% of Poverty
1	$11,880	$13,068	$14,850	$17,820	$20,790	$21,978	$23,760
2	$16,020	$17,622	$20,025	$24,030	$28,035	$29,637	$32,040
3	$20,160	$22,176	$25,200	$30,240	$35,280	$37,297	$40,320
4	$24,300	$26,730	$30,375	$36,450	$42,525	$44,955	$48,600
5	$28,440	$31,284	$35,550	$42,660	$49,770	$52,614	$56,880
6	$32,580	$35,838	$40,725	$48,870	$57,015	$60,273	$65,160
7	$36,730	$40,403	$45,913	$55,095	$64,278	$67,951	$73,460
8	$40,890	$44,979	$51,113	$61,335	$71,558	$75,647	$81,780

The Federal Fiscal Year 2017 guidelines shown here and a family of four at 150 percent of FPG will include households that earn up to $36,450. According to LIHEAP regulations, guarantees can establish the maximum household income for LIHEAP eligibility at either 150 percent of these federal poverty guidelines, or 60 percent of state median income (SMI).

To better help determine eligibility for the *Supplemental Nutrition Assistance Program (SNAP)* and the *Supplemental Security One can use Income Program (SSI)*, as well as other Federal Safety Net Programs such as the 1965 Medicaid or WIC programs. Poverty education has become a major goal for the United Nations and the World Bank, but the U.S, Congress and particularly the conservative Republican Party have done very little over the last ten years to help untangle the confusion. The Far-right Republican conservatives want to privatize these services like health insurance and then transfer the savings to the wealthy faction's .01% instead of what should be a non-profit cost-effective understandable tax supported

Federal program. Doesn't this sound familiar?

Jobs & Exporting Jobs:
The total U.S. nonfarm payroll employment statistic increased by $209,000 in July 2017, according to the *Bureau of Labor Statistics (BLS)*. The unemployed in the U.S. as of January 2013 was 12.3 million persons, and this statistic decreased to 7.5 by the end of 2016. The unemployment rate was 7.9 percent as of January 2013 and decreased to 4.3 percent at the end of 2016 — however; the economy has only gotten worse because today's Multi-party Congress refuses to establish a workable annual budget or adequately represent the people's democracy in a bi-partisan manner. From 1990 to 2015, employment percentage growth has been as follows:

Education	*105%*
Health & Social Services	*99%*
Professional & Business	*81%*
Leisure & Hospitality	*63%*
Transportation & Warehousing	*39%*
Other Services	*32%*
All	*30%*
Financial	*23%*
Construction	*22%*
Government	*20%*
Retail Trade	*19%*
Wholesale Trade	*12%*
Mining & Logging	*7%*
Information	*2%*
Utilities	*-25%*
Manufacturing	*-30%*

The unemployment rate has shown little improvement recently, and among the major worker groups, the unemployment rates for both adult men and women was 4.0 percent, and for teenagers 13.2 percent. The unemployment rate for White workers was 3.8 percent; Blacks 7.4 percent; Asians 3.8 percent; and Hispanics 5.1 percent.

The number of long-term unemployed workers in the U.S. was 1.8 million in July 2017, which comprised 25.9 percent of the unemployed that were jobless for 27 weeks or more. During that same period, there were 5.3

million persons employed part-time for economic reasons, and they were referred to as "Involuntary Part-Time Workers," while 1.6 million persons are *"Marginally Attached Workers,"* not included in the labor force. Marginally Attached Workers were available for work and may have looked for a job during the previous 12 months, and yet they are not counted as unemployed. Within this group, some 536,000 discouraged workers have stopped looking for work because they believed there were no jobs available, and the remaining 1.1 million persons had not even searched for work for reasons such as school attendance or family responsibilities. Job outsourcing is when U.S. companies hire foreign workers instead of Americans, and this increases U.S. Unemployment. Job outsourcing helps almost every U.S. international overseas company to sell to foreign markets, and it helps keep labor costs low where the standards of living are less costly — which hopefully lowers prices on the goods they ship back to the United States. Many foreign employees are hired to help with local marketing, contacts, and language. However, most American workers would not be willing to accept the low wages paid to foreign employees, and if they did, the American consumers would still be forced to pay higher prices. If the U.S. renegotiates NAFTA or imposed higher tariffs that would raise the prices of products made in those countries, it would make it very difficult for American-made goods to compete with cheaper foreign goods. Imposing laws to restrict job outsourcing artificially might lead some companies to move their company overseas, and those that did try to compete at a higher product cost would most likely go out of business.

CNN.Com — previously listed over 800 companies as "Exporting America," by sending American jobs overseas or choosing to employ cheap overseas labor in place of American workers. Competition for low-wage jobs with China and other underdeveloped countries has also driven down salaries in the U.S. for non-college degreed workers, which involves close to 70% (100 million) of the workers in the United States, according to the U.S. Census Bureau. Isolationists would rather see the United States take care of its own, while the profit-seeking NWO continues to distribute jobs across the globe which helps support costly wars, and helps the U.S. to gain greater control over other countries natural resources.

1 William Ripple, Oregon State University, an ecologist

14

Personal Issues

Gun Control:
Gun laws of the United States are in the federal statutes, and these laws regulate the manufacture, trade, possession, transfer, record keeping, transport, and destruction of firearms, ammunition, and all firearms accessories. The *"Bureau of Alcohol, Tobacco, Firearms, and Explosives" (AFT)* enforces these laws. The Second Amendment to the United States Constitution enforces the right for a person to keep and bear firearms. Unfortunately, however, the U.S. has a unique role in both the ownership and use of guns, particularly when compared with other nations. Sadly the violence involving firearms in the U.S. has become far more widespread even though gun ownership in the United States is declining. However, there is an increase in mass killings in the U.S. that includes such mass killings like the twelve people killed in an Aurora, Colorado movie theater — or a gunman killed 27 people, including 20 children, at the Sandy Hook Elementary School in Newton, Connecticut. And then more recently when a gunman killed nine people at a historic African American church in Charleston, S.C. And last, but not least, when Stephen Paddock, a Mesquite resident, killed 58 people and himself after wounding nearly 500 others attending the outdoor Route 91 Harvest Country Music Festival at Las Vegas Village.

U.S. Killings and injuries from 2005 to 2016
FEB. 14, 2018 - 17 killed, 15 injured in Frankland, FL Marjory Stoneman High School by an 18-year-old expelled student Nicholas Cruz.

JUNE 12, 2016 - 50 killed, 53 injured in Orlando nightclub shooting by 29-year-old Omar Mateen.

DEC. 2, 2015 - 14 dead, 22 wounded: San Bernardino, Calif. by U.S.-born Syed Rizwan Farook and Pakistan national Tashfeen Malik.

NOV. 29, 2015 - 3 dead, nine injured: Colorado Springs, Colo. - Robert Lewis Dear.

OCT. 1, 2015 - 9 dead, 9 injured: Roseburg, Ore. by Christopher Sean Harper - who had mental health issues.

JULY 16, 2015 - 5 dead, three wounded: Chattanooga, Tenn. - by Mohammed Youssuf Abdulazeez, 24.

JUNE 18, 2015 - 9 dead: Charleston, S.C. by Emanuel African Methodist Episcopal Church - by Dylann Storm Roof - suspected white supremacist.

MAY 23, 2014 - 6 dead, seven wounded: Isla Vista, California - by Elliot Rodger, 22.

APRIL 2, 2014 - 3 killed, 16 injured: Ft. Hood, Texas - gunman is dead at the scene.

SEPT. 16, 2013 - 12 killed, three injured: Washington, D.C. - by Aaron Alexis - extensive Navy disciplinary record.

JUNE 7, 2013 - 5 killed: Santa Monica - by John Zawahri.

DEC. 14, 2012 - 27 killed, one injured: Newtown, Conn. - Sandy Hook Elementary School in Newtown, Conn. - by Adam Lanza, 20, School.

OCT. 21, 2012 - 3 dead, four injured: Brookfield, Wis. - by Radcliffe Haughton, 45, Public place.

SEPT. 28, 2012 - 6 killed, two injured: Minneapolis, Minn. - by Andrew Engeldinger, 36, Workplace.

AUG. 5, 2012 - 6 killed, three injured: Oak Creek, Wis. - by Wade Michael Page, a white supremacist.

JULY 20, 2012 - 12 killed, 58 injured: Aurora, Colo. - by James Holmes, 24, Public place.

APRIL 2, 2012 - 7 killed, three injured: Oakland - by L. Goh, 43.

OCT. 12, 2011- 8 killed, one injured: Seal Beach, Calif. -by Scott Dekraai, 44, Workplace.

JAN. 8, 2011 - 6 killed, 11 injured: Tucson, Ariz. Shoots Arizona Rep. Gabrielle Giffords - by Jared Lee Loughner, 22, Public place.

AUG. 3, 2010 - 8 killed, two injured: Manchester, Conn. - by Omar S. Thornton, 34, Workplace.

FEB. 12, 2010 - 3 killed, 3 wounded: Huntsville, Ala. - by Amy Bishop, 45, Workplace.

NOV. 5, 2009 - 13 killed, 32 injured: Ft. Hood, Texas - by Maj. Nidal Malik Hasan, an Army psychiatrist.

APRIL 3, 2009 - 13 killed, four injured: Binghamton, N.Y. - by Jiverly Voong, 41, Public place.

FEB. 14, 2008 - 5 killed, 16 injured: Dekalb, Ill. - by Steven Kazmierczak.

DEC. 5, 2007 - 8 killed, four injured: Omaha, NEB. - by Robert Hawkins, 19, Public place.

APRIL 16, 2007 - 32 killed, 17 injured: Blacksburg, Va. - by Seung-hui Cho, 23, School.

FEB. 12, 2007 - 5 killed, four injured: Salt Lake City, Utah - by Sulejman Talovic, 18, Public place.

OCT. 2, 2006 - 5 killed, 5 injured: Nickel Mines, Pa. - by Charles Carl Roberts IV.

JAN. 30, 2006 - 6 dead, Goleta, Calif. - by Jennifer San Marco.

MARCH 21, 2005 - 9 killed, 7 injured: Red Lake Indian Reservation, Minn. - by Jeffrey Weise, a 16-year-old student.

From 1984 to 1994 19 incidents resulted in 155 deaths, while during the assault weapon ban from 1994 to 2004 there were only 12 incidents and 89 deaths. Over the last ten years, Congress has done nothing about the above listed 293 killings and 372 injuries involving guns. A majority of the U.S. population overwhelmingly wants something done as shown by the following nationwide poles.

- *Eighty-five percent of the public supports background checks for private and gun show sales.*
- *Eighty percent of the public supports people with mental illness from purchasing guns.*
- *Sixty-seven of the public support having a Federal database to track gun sales.*
- *Sixty-four percent of the public support having armed security guards and police in more schools.*
- *Fifty-eight percent of the public support a ban on semi-automatic weapons.*
- *Fifty-five percent of the public support a ban on assault-style weapons.*
- *Fifty-four percent of the public support a ban on hi-capacity ammunition clips.*
- *Fifty-three percent of the public support a ban on the online sale of ammunition.*
- *Forty percent of the public supports more teachers and school officials with guns in schools.*

Note: International studies have shown gun policies help lower murders across the globe. Gun killings fell during the assault weapon ban of 1994.

Age:

The *"Age Discrimination in Employment Act (ADEA)"* of 1967 forbids age discrimination against people 40 or older, and it does not protect workers under the age of 40.

Disability:

Disability discrimination occurs when an employer or other entity covered by the *"Americans with Disabilities Act of 1990,"* (amended) — or the *"Rehabilitation Act of 1973,"* (amended) treats a qualified individual with a disability who is an employee or applicant unfavorably because she or he has a disability.

Equal Pay and Compensation:

The *"Equal Pay Act of 1963"* requires that men and women receive equal pay for equal work. The job's content (not titles) determines whether jobs are equal. Pay covered by this law, including salary, overtime pay, bonuses, stock options, profit sharing, and bonus plans, life insurance, vacation and holiday pay, cleaning or gasoline allowances, hotel accommodations, reimbursement for travel expenses, and the employers may not reduce the wages of either sex to equalize their pay.

Genetic Information:

Genetic information dealing with genetic discrimination in employment includes information about an employee's genetic tests or any individual's family member's tests documented in any family member's medical history involving the manifestation of a disease or disorder. The *"Equal Employment Opportunity Commission (EEOC) of 1965"* enforces *"Title II of the Genetic Information Nondiscrimination Act (GINA)."* The *"Departments of Labor, Health and Human Services and the Treasury"* having responsibility for issuing regulations for *"Title I of GINA,"* which addresses the use of genetic information in health insurance.

Harassment:

Harassment is a form of employment discrimination that violates *"Title VII"* of the *Civil Rights Act of 1964*, the *"Age Discrimination in Employment Act of 1967, (ADEA),"* and the *"Americans with Disabilities Act of 1990, (ADA)."* Harassment is unwelcome conduct based on race, color, religion, sex (including pregnancy), national origin, age 40 or older, disability or genetic information. Anti-discrimination laws also prohibit harassment.

Harassment becomes unlawful where:

- *Enduring the offensive conduct becomes a condition of continued employment, or*

- *The conduct is severe or pervasive enough to create a work environment that a reasonable person would consider intimidating, hostile, or abusive.*

National Origin:

The *"National Origin Discrimination Act of 1964"* involves treating employees or applicants for a job unfavorably because they are from a particular country or part of the world, because of ethnicity or accent, or because they appear to be of certain ethnic background. The law forbids discrimination when it comes to any aspect of employment, including hiring, firing, pay, job assignments, promotions, layoff, training, fringe benefits, and any other term or condition of employment.

Pregnancy:

The *"Pregnancy Discrimination Act (PDA) of 1978"* is a United States federal statute. *"Title VII of the Civil Rights Act of 1964"* (amended) to prohibit sex discrimination by pregnancy, which involved treating a woman employee or applicant for a job unfavorably because of pregnancy, childbirth, or a medical condition related to pregnancy or childbirth. The PDA forbids discrimination based on pregnancy when it comes to any aspect of employment, including hiring, firing, pay, job assignments, promotions, layoff, training, fringe benefits, such as leave and health insurance, and any other term or condition of employment.

Race or Color:

The *"Race Relations Act of 1965"* involves treating an employee or applicant for a job unfavorably because he/she is of a certain race or because of personal characteristics associated with race such as hair texture, skin color, or certain facial features. People have been immigrating to the U.S. from all around the world for centuries, but millions of Africans brought to the US by force were held in slavery. Blacks were forced to come to the U.S. as slaves, creating considerable discrimination and it is amazing how well the black race has handled this in that they now excel in many arts that particularly involve music, dancing, voice, sports, acting, news media, and civil rights issues. The various racial and color groups discriminated against in the U.S. are African Americans, Hispanics,

Asians, Muslims, Jews, and other immigrant groups such as the Lesbian, Gay, Bisexual, and Transgender (LGBT) community. The Republican Congress and the President, have allowed the topic of illegal immigration to once again rise to the forefront of American politics. As a result, *Racial Intolerance, (Xenophobia)*, which is the intense and irrational dislike or fear of people from other countries, is on the rise. Because of this, the nation is once again becoming divided and confused on both racial issues and what to do about the millions of illegal immigrants currently living on American soil. And now this President intends to build a wall that will prevent any illegal Mexican immigrants from crossing the border. Illegal profiling is once again being used to question the legal status of anyone that even looks foreign. It's gotten so bad that Americans are confused with Muslim by their dress or outward appearance, which is causing discrimination amongst U.S. citizens. And with all of the financial instability in the U.S. economy today, many Americans believe their jobs are in jeopardy

Racial Issues:
Most of today's racial standards were developed back in the 1960s when by-partisan decisions were still possible before today's Multi-party liberal and conservative issues brought this nation to a standstill.

Religion:
"Title VII" of the *"Civil Rights Act"* and the *"Religious Freedom Restoration Act (RFRA) of 1964"* prohibits employers from engaging in religious discrimination in the workplace. Religious discrimination involves treating an employee or an applicant for a job unfavorably because of his or her religious beliefs. The law protects not only people who belong to traditional organized religions, such as Muslim, Buddhism, Christianity, Hinduism, Islam, and Judaism as well as others who hold religious, ethical or moral beliefs.

Retaliation:
The *"U.S. Equal Employment Opportunity Commission (EEOC) of 1965"* involved the federal agency that administers and enforces civil rights laws against workplace discrimination. This Commission's laws prohibit punishing employees or an applicant for a job unfavorably or asserting their rights to be free from employment discrimination, including

harassment. Asserting these EEO rights is called *"protected activity,"* and it can take many forms. For example, it is unlawful to retaliate against applicants or employees for:

- *Filing or being a witness to an EEO charge, complaint, investigation, or lawsuit.*
- *For communicating with management about employment discrimination and harassment.*
- *Answering questions during an employer investigation of alleged harassment.*
- *Refusing to follow orders that would result in discrimination.*
- *Resisting sexual advances, or intervening to protect others.*
- *For Requesting accommodation for a disability or religious practice.*
- *Requesting salary information involving discriminatory wages.*

Sex:
The *"Sex Discrimination Act of 1975"* involves treating an employee or an applicant for a job unfavorably because of that person's sex. The law forbids discrimination when it comes to any aspect of employment, including hiring, firing, pay, job assignments, promotions, layoff, training, fringe benefits, and any other term or condition of employment.

Sexual Harassment:
"Sexual Harassment" since 1970, holds that it is unlawful to harass an employee or an applicant for a job because of that person's sex. Harassment can include any form of sexual harassment or unwelcome sexual advances, requests for sexual favors, and other verbal or physical harassment of a sexual nature. Harassment does not have to be sexual and can include offensive remarks about a person's sex. For example, it is illegal to harass a woman by making offensive comments about women in general. Both the victim and the harasser can be either a woman or a man.

Mental Illness, Drug, Alcoholism, Vagrancy:
In 1977, the St. Joseph's hospital in Lansing, Michigan and the Michigan State Medical School under Dr. William Knisely, obtained a Federal Grant to establish a Regional Mental Health Center in Lansing, Michigan. They built the center and staffed the center under a leading psychiatrist by the name of Dr. Allen Enlow. Just before opening this Michigan, Illinois,

Indiana three state regional mental health center, the Conservative Republican President, Richard Nixon, withdrew the funding as a budgetary measure that forced the mentally ill and drug-addicted patients back out on the streets. Nixon's decision filled the jails and prisons as it shattered any future professional solution to this country's mental illness, drug, alcoholism, and vagrancy problems. The Cook County Jail in Chicago recently hired a Psychiatrist to serve as the Warden to try to better handle this Jail's mentally ill and drug population, which currently constitutes almost 50% of the prison's population nationally. This financial approach versus a clinical approach has frustrated the medical profession who takes an oath to *"Do no Harm."* The U.S. Congress has intentionally ping-ponged this nation's sick and disabled in and out of proper care while forcing them to pay a profit *to the profit-seeking insurance and pharmaceutical industries* so politicians can receive benefits for corporate favors.

15

Policing Other Nations

The United States of America should maintain a strong military, but the U.S. can no longer afford to police the world or continue to provide foreign aid at the rate the U.S. has in the past. The UN should and could be responsible for policing the world, if not controlled by the TC and the CFR. With the national debt currently growing exponentially, and the cost of maintaining U.S. military bases, which are seven times greater than any other nation, perhaps it's time to change direction. We continue to borrow almost two million dollars every hour as the Congress eats up well over 50% of the nation's annual discretionary spending budget. The total military spending in the U.S. exceeds the military spending of China, Russia, Japan, and India combined, currently constituting almost half of all the military spending in the entire world. Do the citizens of the U.S. even consider the fact that one F 22 Fighter jet cost this nation 360 million dollars, and we currently maintain military bases in more than 130 nations throughout the world? Worse yet, policing other nations is no longer gaining friends. This country's unjust wars in Iraq and Afghanistan alone have cost the U.S. working class more than a trillion dollars of their hard earned tax dollars while costing every individual taxpayer in the U.S. between three to four thousand dollars a year. On top of all that, this country's politicians continue to try and persuade us that foreign aid helps the giver more than the receiver, but we all know that is no longer true. The U.S. planes bomb Afghanistan, Iraq, Pakistan, Libya, Yemen, and Somalia and it seems that the more the U.S. bombs, the more these countries, and the entire world hates us, and in addition to North Korea, a growing number of them now openly say they want to destroy the United States. And to be honest, the U.S. is creating far more enemies than we're destroying. With terrorists everywhere, it's time for the U.S. to find a different way to solve the terrorist problems. On top of this, the U.S. can no longer afford the cost of war when this nation is financially on the verge of a huge depression. And yet this nation's wealthy faction is seeking more money by supporting wars with Iran, Syria and North Korea. Every American already knows that any conflict with terrorists requires something other than a powerful military force, or a nuclear war with North Korea. It's getting well past the time where the U.S. citizens will soon have to demand a change in the direction this dysfunctional Congress has been heading.

After viewing several government reports on U.S. Foreign Aid, we can now fairly accurately determine that the U.S. spent more than fifty-two billion on foreign aid in the fiscal year following this nation's 2008 depression, of which more than thirty-two billion was for economic aid, and fifteen billion was for military aid. The top 25 countries that were the recipients of this U.S Foreign Aid included:

Afghanistan, Pakistan, Israel, Iraq, Egypt, Haiti, Ethiopia, Sudan, Columbia, Kenya, Jordan, Mexico, Senegal, West Bank/ Gaza, South Africa, Tanzania, Russia, Nigeria, Georgia, Mozambique, Congo (Kinshasa), Indonesia, and Zambia, Kazakhstan

Although the aid the U.S. provides is now often referred to as *"buying off other countries"* — this needs to be reviewed in greater detail because the implications of providing this human service are far too costly. Since this type of Foreign Aid is thought to be a tool to gain influence over developing countries, it has also had an enormous political implication. The U.S. was first forced to provide Foreign Aid when the 1913 bankers took control of the Federal Reserve and their Multilateral Development Banks (MDB) that saw this as a tremendous loan advantage for themselves and their international corporations in gaining greater control over the developing country's businesses and their natural resources. Although the *"Trilateral Commission (TLC)"* and the *"Council on Foreign Relations (CFR)"* were responsible for writing the By-Laws and Articles of Incorporation of the UN, this MDB selfishly sought to control the business income and the natural resources of these developing countries. The U.S. has now become involved in a growing battle with China who seeks personal and financial gain through their bank loans from the

"Multilateral Development Banks (MDBs)," the *"World Bank,"* or the *"Asian Development Bank (ADB)"* and the *"Inter-American Development Banks (IDB)."*

If foreign aid had originally started under a functional type UN organization, it might have had a far better chance of providing such human services to the entire world without profit and control over a country's natural resources being the primary goal of today's foreign aid program. As a result, the U.S. has created a constant and growing conflict with China — a conflict that we are losing, as well as an ongoing battle between two superpowers that will find it very difficult ever to resolve peacefully. Chinese foreign aid has more recently been growing rapidly in comparison to the U.S., and it is becoming very noticeable that the Chinese government can wield considerable influence over a growing number of communist oriented developing nations, thereby rapidly advancing they're communist strategic and economic goals and objectives. The *"BRICS,"* include Brazil, Russia, India, China, and South Africa, which is a group of five major emerging economies that seek to reform the United Nations and implement tougher measures against terrorist groups. The BRICS recently denounced North Korea's nuclear tests at a summit in China, seeking to enlarge their presence on the world stage.

In other words, Chinese foreign aid undercuts the U.S. goals, such as this nation's desire to promote democratic governance through developmental aid, while also advancing global markets and economic reform. Some of the issues this duality of aid to other countries creates include:

- *It offers a source for competitive Communist regimes to cost-effectively fund their infrastructure and humanitarian needs*

- *It allows the Chinese to support regimes with poor human rights records*

- *It opens the door for China to focus their assistance on their own economic need to expand their access to oil, gas, and other natural resources that are already at a serious shortage, as well as competitively marketing Chinese products.*

- *As a part of any Chinese aid contract, the recipient countries must adhere to diplomatic loyalty to China on the political issue the United States has with*

China, such as on Taiwan, Tibet and the many more controversial concerns between so many countries.

- *Both China and the U.S. also seek greater influence in the Multilateral Development Banks (MDB's), such as the World Bank, since China also uses the MDB's to provide investment assistance to developing countries.*

Fortunately, the U.S. still holds the dominant shareholding power by controlling over 16 percent of the voting power in the *"World Bank's International Bank for Reconstruction and Development (IBRD)"* while China controls just under, 5 percent. And in the (ADB) the U.S. again controls almost 16 percent of shareholder voting power while China currently controls a little more than 6 percent. The U.S. also controls some 30 percent of the voting power in the *"IDB"* while China controls less than one percent, which gives the U.S. temporary advantage over the voting power of the MDB's, but there is a question of how long this will last under the U.S.'s very shaky financial condition. Another very serious problem involves the foreign aid countries (such as Pakistan) that are seeing U.S. money going directly into the pockets of their wealthy power factions with less of the U.S donations used for the aid intended. Therefore, as Congress determines its budget priorities, the effectiveness of funding foreign aid requires far greater scrutiny regarding the fact that the current programs may not be accomplishing the goals originally intended. The way today's dysfunctional Congress responds to this problem will influence U.S. foreign policy for years to come. In that foreign aid has been a huge financial and political drain on the U.S., it appears this nation will eventually have no choice but to discontinue this program and let China pursue this role until they eventually reach that same conclusion the U.S. is now reaching. Although some of the programs are important human services, the human service of aiding the development of other countries must eventually fall to the UN because the U.S. can no longer expect its working class to add to its already financial breaking budget that is well on its way to destroying the U.S. democracy through bankruptcy. Wouldn't it be nice if the U.S. sought to cure cancer or provide universal comprehensive health care cost-free to the sick and disabled throughout the world, or solve the many environmental problems that are about to destroy the human race?

16

International Concerns

The *"International Law Commission (ILC)"* is an appointed body of legal experts appointed by the UN's General Assembly, that in 1994 established a permanent international criminal court. By 1996, the ILC defined the crimes against the peace and security of humanity, which reflected the UN's agreement that an international criminal court, with a fair trial for the accused, should be created to accomplish a more just world under the rule of law. After years of not having an established International Criminal Court with jurisdiction to try war crimes and crimes against humanity, it was finally accomplished and formally approved in 1998 by the UN after the required number of nation's ratified it. As a result, the ILC holds the hope of putting an end to the lack of punishment for world crimes against humanity — thereby creating a legally humane and just world, if the controlling CFR will allow this to happen.

David Rockefeller served as the Director Emeritus (Honorary Chairman) of the CFR, which the Rockefeller's Foundation funded and incorporated in 1921. This private CFR involved Colonel House, JP Morgan, John D Rockefeller, Paul Warburg, Otto Kahn, and Jacob Schiff, the very same U.S. appointed commission that had, under considerable controversy, created this nation's privately held Federal Reserve System in 1913. The CFR is an independent foreign policy membership organization that built the UN building on land donated by David Rockefeller. David Rockefeller sent close to fifty CFR members to the UN's 1929 initial meeting in San Francisco, where these very powerful and wealthy individuals of the world were able to influence the initial drafting of the future charter for the UN. Such control was necessary so the CFR could replace the U.S.'s leadership role it had taken on after World War II, thereby allowing the wealthy faction to better protect their wealth under their control — instead of being under a U.S. Democracy that sought equality for all. The *"UN Conference on International Organizations"* met later in San Francisco on the 25th of April, 1945 to finalize the drafting of the UN Charter supported by a proper number of governments — while the CFR negotiated with the Allied Big Four, which included the Soviet Union, the UK, China, and the U.S.

David Rockefeller, the undisputed *"Overlord"* of his family's corporate monopoly, was also one of the founders of the *"Trilateral Commission"* (TC), which was also his brainchild. The TC was a non-government discussion group he founded in July 1973 to foster closer cooperation among the Tri-Lats, which initially included North America, Western Europe, and Japan. David Rockefeller first developed the idea of the TC at one of their family meetings at his Pocantico Hills estate just outside of New York City with the underlying intention of leveling the U.S. to the same level as other nations. The U.S. had become far too powerful for the CSR to aggressively seek total control over the *"World Market,"* the *"International Industrial Complex,"* and this nation's *"Armed Services."* The CFR intentionally ignored *"International Laws,"* that would control their decision making.

The Rockefellers have had a long history of being heavily involved in funding and supporting numerous wealthy and powerful organizations like the *"Bilderberger's"* they incorporated on May 29th, 1954 in Knokke, Belgium. John D. Rockefeller Sr. (July 8, 1839 – May 23, 1937) was a monopolist who hated competition and always sought control of his investments. Therefore his son David became actively involved in the Bilderbergers, which meets annually at a private conference involving some 150 European, North American, and Japanese members. These members are international financiers, industrialists, media magnates, union bosses, academics, and political figures whose countries all belong to the *"North Atlantic Treaty Organization (NATO)"* established in April 1949. NATO 's located in Brussels, Belgium, which once served as a western countermeasure against aggression by the Soviet Union during the Cold War.

Another area that requires International Law being spelled out in writing is what has happened to the world banks as a result of the U.S. Federal Reserve Act that was unwillingly passed by the U.S. Congress in 1913. At that time, the people of the U.S. Democracy were not aware that a world banking system was being set up by the powerful international bankers, or the wealthy faction and international industrialists that intended to control the world's financial system.

Peter Kershaw, in his book, *"Economic Solutions"* identifies the U.S. IRS as the *"collection agency"* for these multinational bank owners — recommending the U.S. citizens petition to repeal the Federal Reserve Act and the IRS code. He also identified the major shareholders of the Federal Reserve Bank System as:

> *Rothschild (London and Berlin)*
> *Lazard Brothers (Paris)*
> *Israel Seiff (Italy)*
> *Kuhn - Loeb Company (Germany)*
> *Warburg (Hamburg and Amsterdam)*
> *Lehman Brothers (New York)*
> *Goldman and Sachs (New York)*
> *Rockefeller (New York)*

This takeover by this wealthy faction has now gained control over the *"Alt-Right Republican Congress"* and helped to establish many other pervasive organizations that have become members of the *"Tri-Lats."* It's important *"We the People"* identify these growing pervasive organizations, which currently control much of this nation's dysfunctional Congress — which is causing the U.S. economy and *"We the People"* to grow weak, while the world becomes more fearful and unfriendly. Here are some of the more important organizations that are seeking to replace the once powerful U.S. Democracy:

> The Trilateral Commission (TC)
> The Bilderbergers
> The Council on Foreign Relations (CFR)
> The North Atlantic Treaty Organization (NATO)
> The North American Free Trade Agreement (NAFTA)
> The American Legislative Exchange Council (ALEC)

The U.S. Federal Reserve
The International Investment Banks and Corporations
The current CFR controlled United Nations (UN)
The American Israel Public Affairs Committee (AIPAC's)
The World Constitution and Parliament Association (WCPA)

Perhaps with today's duly elected U.S. Congress rendered so dysfunctional by so many outside benefits and favors — these monopolistic organizations are having a far greater influence over this sovereign nation and its working class. Perhaps the U.S. citizens should have determined what they wanted before they let all these *"Kleptocratic Aristocracies"* take over this nation's Democracy under what will inevitably become a powerful multinational fascist controlled system.

The **"TC"** meets behind closed doors every year, making decisions for the U.S. Congress. David Rockefeller ran the *"Manhattan Bank,"* and later served as the CEO of the service arm of *"JP Morgan Chase."* He is the undisputed *"Overlord"* and founder of the TC. The TC is intended to be the vehicle for multinational consolidation of the commercial and banking interests, thereby gaining control over the U.S government.

Barry Goldwater said:
"The TC is international and is intended to be the vehicle for multinational consolidation of the commercial and banking interests by seizing control of the political government of the United States. The Trilateral Commission represents a skillful, coordinated effort to seize control and consolidate the four centers of power – political, monetary, intellectual and ecclesiastical."(1)

Then in 1994, the **"North American Free Trade Agreement (NAFTA)"** was proposed to create the world's largest free trade zone that would allow strong economic growth in Canada, the United States, and Mexico, but here again, little was done to define the standards that would be required. They sought to remove standards that had become a barrier to the exchange of goods and services among the three countries.

Author Molly Ivins who coined the word "Shrub" in the "Shrub Dynasty" to identify George H.W. Bush's job with the CIA and his close ties with the CFR posed a serious concern for this nation's Democracy.

Admiral Chester Ward, a former member and unsympathetic critic of the CFR, states in his book: "Kissinger on the Couch."

> *"The most powerful cliques in these elitist groups have one objective in common: they want to bring about the surrender of the sovereignty and national independence of the United States."(2)*

And as all Americans know, President Kennedy never had a chance to do that.

On December 2, 2017, the Majority Republican Senate ignored the Democrats and the people and unilaterally accepted the CFR as the major benefactor in their taxation proposal. Trickle-down economics has previously not worked, and the Bush recession placed the wealthy faction of the CFR under a spotlight that proved to be very embarrassing. Financiers suggest the current Republican Senate proposal is almost certainly going to substantially increase the deficit by an estimated ten trillion dollars over the next ten years. Some 400 fearful American millionaires and billionaires sent a letter to the Senate in November 2017, urging them not to cut their taxes, and this was because they do not like being placed in the spotlight as the ones who are behind the destruction of the greatest Democracy in the world. These wealthy entrepreneurs letter called upon Congress not to pass any tax bill that:

> *"further exasperates inequality and would add to the debt"* while it even called for *"Congress to raise taxes on the rich."*

However, the unilateral Republican proposal was still passed knowing that it will add $1.5 trillion to the deficit the very first year the tax proposal goes into effect. But if the Republicans had not accomplished this, they would receive no bonus for the many favors they bestow on the CFR members.

The **International Investment Banks and Corporations** that hold membership in the Tri-Lats comprises a large number of the most powerful *"full-service global investment banks"* that provide advisory and financing banking services, as well as sales, marketing, and research on a broad array of financial products — including equities, credit, rates, currency, commodities, and derivatives. This includes the following banks:

> *The JP Morgan Chase; Goldman Sachs; Bank of America; Merrill Lynch; Morgan Stanly; Citigroup; Barclays Investment Bank; Credit Suisse; Deutsche Bank; Wells Fargo Securities; RBC Capital Markets; UBS, HSBC; Jefferies Group; BNP Paribas; Mizuho; Lazard; Nomura; Evercore Partners; BMO Capital Markets; Mitsubishi UFJ Financial Group.*

The current dysfunctional **UN** also has yet to prove they are free from CFR control.

The **American Israel Public Affairs Committee (AIPAC's)**

In going to war with Iraq, America inadvertently chose to support the neoconservatives and the U.S. alliance with Israel, the *"American Israel Public Affairs Committee (AIPAC)"* and their Likud-Zionist Prime Minister, Ariel Sharon, which generated a new frontier of worldwide anti-Americanism and anti-semitic bigotry of global proportions. Predictably, the U.S. Isreal alliance occurred with little or no understanding of the complex conflict that was raging between Judaism and Zionism — specifically concerning the religious, racial, and ethnic issues that were disrupting the entire Muslim and European cultures throughout the entire world. Here are some of the deceitful lies proposed by this nation's neoconservative leaders:

- *Iraq is reconstituting its nuclear weapons. (10/07/02)*

- *Saddam Hussein is seeking quantities of uranium from Africa. (10/28/03)*

- *Saddam has reconstituted nuclear weapons. (03/16/03)*

- *The CIA has solid reporting of senior-level contacts between Iraq and al-Qaeda going back a decade. (10/07/02)*

- *Iraq has trained al-Qaeda members in bomb-making and poisons and deadly gases, and their alliances with terrorists could allow Iraq to attack America. (10/07/02)*

- *Iraq has a growing fleet of manned and unmanned aerial vehicles that could disperse chemical or biological weapons. (10/07/02)*

- *We have seen intelligence over many months that Iraq has dispersed chemical and biological weapons, and that command control arrangements have been established. (02/08/03)*

- *Conservative estimates are that Iraq has a stockpile of between 100 and 500 tons of chemical weapons agents to fill some 16,000 rockets. (02/05/02)*

- *Iraq's WMD are, located around Tikrit and Baghdad and east, south, and north somewhat. (03/30/03)*

- *We found a biological laboratory in Iraq, which the UN prohibited. (06/01/03)*

- *Blaming Iraq for the Trade Center destruction*

The destruction involving the *"World Trade Center"* demanded some immediate form of retaliation by the U.S., but it was irresponsible for the U.S. to add to the problem between Judaism and Zionism by starting an unjustified war in Iraq. The Iraq war disrupted its many neighboring states that included Iran, Afghanistan, Turkey, Libya, Syria, Lebanon, Jordan, Egypt, Saudi Arabia, and Germany and France. Iran now controls the Shiite population in both Iran and Iraq, and many of these countries blame the resulting religious war in Iraq on the U.S., called the *"Rapture"* or the *"Apocalyptic Event,"* in which God will destroy the ruling powers of evil. In other words, these countries believe that all these suicidal terrorist bombings we see are on behalf of God — and that these protagonists will go to heaven in an unending war that culminates with the end of the earth. Most of the world, outside of the U.S. now recognizes the Iraqi war was not a matter of *"win or lose,"* and are now realizing that it was a huge neoconservative contrived mistake for this nation to ignore the real terrorist, Al Qaeda's Osama bin Laden. How could the U.S. have been so stupid as to authorize a unilateral act of aggression without a clear understanding of the facts?

The decision to go to war may have helped G.W. Bush in his re-election, but in Richard Pearl and co-author Douglas Feith's book, "*A Clean Break: A New Strategy for Securing the Realm,*" it promoted the Iraq war. Based on this book, the Israeli Prime Minister, Netanyahu, gave his approval for war long before the Trade Center's destruction in New York. This book called for the elimination of Israel's enemy "Saddam Hussein," and the September 13, 1993 "Oslo Accord," which defined the interim self-government arrangements between the *"Palestinian Liberation Organization (PLO)"* and Israel. It proposed to install a Hashemite monarchy in Baghdad to destabilize the governments of Syria, Lebanon, Saudi Arabia, and Iran, thereby recommending a regional dominance by Israel over that entire area, referred to as *"The Greater Israel,"* which was to become the sole power in the Middle East. The United States and Israel played a major role in this unjust aggression in Iraq and approved without the support of any of the neighboring countries, the UN, or the Muslims estimated to be between 1.2 to 1.4 billion people in the world's almost seven billion population.

Note: Pulling out of the Iran Agreement will most likely prompt another war between Syria and Iran and the U.S., thereby extending the U.S.'s President's term of office.

Since the start of the Iraq war, the United States has and continues to spend trillions of dollars instead of the Bush projected $50 to $80 billion to fight this war that promoted *"Greater Israel."* And more recently, Israel continues to defiantly and intentionally escalate its perpetual religious conflict with Lebanon and Jerusalem. As a result, no one can currently resolve this dangerous Zionist Israeli conflict with Judaism that the U.S. inadvertently encouraged throughout the entire Islamic world — as well as the anti-Americanism and anti-Semitism that has been on the rise throughout the Middle East, Germany, France, and more recently the entire world.

The World Constitution and Parliament Association (WCPA) has been trying to define what a Democracy is, and if one studies their effort, it truly appears to be an impossible task. The greatest democracy in the history of the world is about to fail after 243 years because the growing enemy within has determined that they can best protect their wealth under a fascist system. The U.S. is attempting to provide equality for all but has missed the mark in so many areas that it can never claim that it has created a government of the people, by the people, or for the people. Yes, this government is failing in integration; taxing its citizens equally and fairly; reverting to a dysfunctional Multi-party Congress, that can potentially destroy this amazing democratic constitution that's still only in its infancy. This great democracy has waged war against what has been an amazing effort to establish a *"Democracy"* in place of a winner takes all system. But unless the people of the U.S. are willing to rise as one, compare the facts with what is happening, and then violently repel the enemy in one voice, the U.S is about to fail.

Another very important area that requires proper enforcement of International Law is the horrible profit-seekers tax avoidance scheme promoted by the wealth-seekers and the international corporations. Here again, this involves the very important UN's ILC where nations can once again seek tax stability for every participating UN democracy. These wealth-seekers have successfully been able to hide from the public until recently when their huge profits and ridiculous tax reductions were exposed.

Although the industrial advancements of the twentieth century have been many, the numerous acts of mass violence during this same period are so many that it's hard to comprehend. According to some estimates, nearly 170 million civilians have experienced genocide, war crimes, and crimes against humanity during this recent period in history. The two World Wars lead the U.S. citizens to pledge *"never again"* would the U.S. allow anything similar to occur. The numerous shocking acts of the Nazis were not isolated incidents, which the world has since relegated to history. In just the second half of the twentieth century, millions of people were tortured and killed in the following countries:

> *Russia; Cambodia; Vietnam; Sierra Leone; Chile; the Philippines; the Congo; Bangladesh; Uganda; Iraq; Indonesia; East Timor; El Salvador; Burundi; Argentina; Somalia; Chad; Yugoslavia; and Rwanda.*

But what is even more concerning is the UN and the entire population, meaning the entire world community, witnessed these massacres and passively stood by and done nothing. What's even more frightening is that in almost every case in history, there is a dictator, president, head of state, or military leader that had been responsible for carrying out these atrocities. Not until the world was shocked by the ethnic cleansing in the former Yugoslavia and the genocide in Rwanda, did the UN finally take action. Nations that had previously been unwilling to intervene or block the carnage finally recognized that some action was necessary. So for the first time since Nuremberg, a new international criminal tribunal was hurriedly put in place on an ad hoc basis by the UN Security Council. Finally, under the impetus of increasing concern, it became possible for the UN to draft the model for an *"International Criminal Tribunal"* for Yugoslavia. The international leadership and the wealthy faction that created the UN had been very reluctant to enforce this international criminal law because that could weaken their control. The ILC's predecessors were primarily the Nuremberg and the International Criminal Tribunal for Yugoslavia that had created this concern. However, these tribunals were merely institutions for what was called *"victor's justice."* However, these tribunals did lay the groundwork for the international criminal law under the UN's ILC. In fact, the ILC's statutes have created the first tribunals where violators of international law can now be held responsible for their crimes. These tribunals also rejected historically used defenses based on state sovereignty, by a resolution made by the UN's General Assembly.

Hopefully, the UN's ILC will soon be tested regarding North Korea's nuclear threat if the current President of the U.S. does not cause a third World War before the ILC can take the necessary steps to bring this nuclear threat to an end in both North Korea and Iran.

The Nuremberg trials attempted to establish the fact that all humanity should be under an international legal organization where criminals and even heads of state can be held criminally responsible for *"Crimes against Humanity"* — now confirmed in writing by the UN's ILC written statutes. However, enforcing proper Democratic principles and standards may still be delayed by the powerful CFR factions that still control the UN, the U.S. Congress, the U.S. tax, and budget system, and the U.S. Federal Reserve, while promoting the off-shore-tax evasion system.

1 Barry Goldwater speech
2 Admiral Chester Ward, in his book: "Kissinger On The Couch."

SECTION III

Having read the facts about the current U.S. political situation, it's important that the U.S. citizen make their own decisions if this greatest Democracy ever hopes to recover the freedom they've unknowingly lost to the powerful Cartel during the Twentieth Century's technical revolution.

Making Your Decisions

Having reviewed the facts about the current U.S. political situation, it's important that the U.S. citizens vote by popular vote before or by the next election to amend the three major mistakes made during the twentieth century, which are currently preventing the people from ever taking back their Democracy. There is almost no way this greatest Democracy can recover the freedom they've unknowingly lost to this powerful Business and Bankers Cartel, the current Dysfunctional Duopoly Multi-Party Congress, and the world's failed effort at Globalization without amending the Constitution and the Declaration of Independence. Next, every citizen needs to make their own decisions to resolve what's been happening to the U.S. Your decisions may not be the same as others, but it's important you find your voice and then use it.

Facts to remember:

- This Cartel's Federal Reserve Banking System is not subject to oversight by either the U.S. Congress or the President.

- Incorporating the "Council of Foreign Relations (CFR), was a major step toward an international takeover of the greatest democracy in the history of the world, and in doing so, the CFR took the first step in their planned control of the world market.

- These international banking entrepreneurs had to first gain financially by making large war loans. For example, these entrepreneurs financed a twenty-five million dollar U.S. deficit for World War I, and this Cartel of banks also additionally financed some twenty-two wars during the twentieth - century.

- The Great Depression had caused many of these very wealthy factions and international corporations to question the foundation of this nation's Democracy — considering Fascism, Socialism, and Communism as alternatives that would give them greater control over their wealth, rather than provide equality for every U.S. citizen.

- Today, this Cartel's worldwide power faction continues to aggressively seek total control over the *"World Market,"* the *"International Industrial Complex,"* the *"U.S, Congress,* as well as this nation's *"Armed Services."*

- This country's current spiraling debt of $21.97 trillion, as of December 31, 2018, is largely due to the high-interest rate Americans currently pay the Federal Reserve through their current tax dollars.

- One percent of the U.S. population controls more wealth than the entire U.S. Population, which demands we get money out of politics and once again hold every citizen's rights as sacred.

- It was after the 1812 British war when the U.S. first established the "Era of Good Feelings" by implementing a single political party to replace Andrew Jackson's Democratic party and Henry Clay's Republican Whig party.

- Remember that this nation has once again, grown into an unworkable dysfunctional Democratic and Republican Multi-party Congress that has used the Electoral College to split the people over the last three Presidential terms.

- Remember that the Republican President, and the House and Senate Majority are currently embarrassing the U.S. by destroying the world-wide reputation of this once most highly respected Democracy.

- Remember that the current Majority Party professes to be conservative while favoring the wealthy upper one percent faction so they can receive financial benefits for the many favors they grant the wealthy and the international corporations.

- All citizens should have the right to *"equally"* receive universal healthcare, education, protection from wars — as well as selected infrastructure benefits and other human services paid for by this nation's cost savings non-profit tax-supported systems.

- Globalization of both Democracies and Communist countries are incompatible. In other words, we cannot mix the two into one happy compatible world where everybody gets along with each other. The loss of trillions of dollars in illegal offshore tax havens for the wealthy does not mix with equality for people.

Chapter 2
House and Senate

Questions the Reader Needs to Answer:

- Should we reduce the 535 unsupervised and overstaffed Senate and House of Representatives' members that are costing just under four trillion in wasted Federal Tax dollars? □ Yes □ No □ Don't Know

- Should the U.S. government transfer the current Congresses' federal tax dollars to the state? □ Yes □ No □ Don't Know

- Should *"We the People"* create a *"State Officer's Compensation Commission (SOCC)"* composed of eight to twelve members elected by the people from the various state districts? If so, should each state employ a trained administrator to represent the SOCC board and to prepare, manage, and guide each federal and state appointee under proper people defined congressional policies and standards?
□ Yes □ No □ Don't Know

- Should this administrator oversee each Congress member's approved budget for staff and office expense under the authority of a SOCC board? □ Yes □ No □ Don't Know

- Should the current Congressional benefit programs be replaced with the same health care and related benefits that Congress has authorized for every U.S. citizen, thereby changing the current U.S. House and Senate healthcare and retirement benefit programs to Medicare and Medicaid, and Social Security? □ Yes □ No □ Don't Know

- Should the U.S. end the COLA and all Civil Service perks that these Congressmen receive? □ Yes □ No □ Don't Know

- Should all Congressional appointments be required to take only one single "Oath of Office" with the understanding their job is a privilege and requires they work full-time for the job they were hired to do to earn their salary and not receive financial benefits from some self-serving wealthy plutocrat or corporation lobbyist?
  □ Yes □ No □ Don't Know

- Should all appointed House Members be allowed to serve no more than six, two-year terms, and Senate Members no more than two six-year terms? □ Yes □ No □ Don't Know

- It is because of this lack of organization, all salary and benefit decisions have been left to be made solely by the Congressmen themselves. Should state Senators and House of Representatives that are all appointed by their state be financially supported by the U.S. Office of Personnel Management, which eliminates any form of line authority? □ Yes □ No □ Don't Know

- Should "We the People" stop all outside donations for any Congress Member's re-election, requiring each state to provide reasonable and equal re-election campaign tax dollars to those Congressmen that qualify to seek re-election? □ Yes □ No □ Don't Know

- Should all candidates for re-election no longer receive any outside financial donations or benefits from such organizations as Citizens United, Super "Pacs," or "Cyber" type assistance from any country, corporation, or organization? □ Yes □ No □ Don't Know

- Should the U.S. get all outside money out of politics?
  □ Yes □ No □ Don't Know

- Should the citizens of each state manage their state Congressmen and seek to reduce the unbelievable budget that the Federal Government currently pays to all U.S. Congressmen? □ Yes □ No □ Don't Know

- Should outside donations to the state be accepted to help finance the added cost of the re-election program? □ Yes □ No □ Don't Know

- Because of the constant bickering and lack of trust between the two Multi-parties, where they can't even meet in the same room — should the U.S. amend the Consitution by returning to one single people party? □ Yes □ No □ Don't Know

- Should five hundred and thirty-five Members of Congress become one-hundred with the hope of eventually reducing all state-appointed U.S. Senate and House members to one state member for each? □ Yes □ No □ Don't Know

- Should each State be allowed to appoint one *"local state legislative member"* per each state's designated number of counties, allowing them to become full-time within the districts they represent, where they are in direct contact with the local people that appointed them? □ Yes □ No □ Don't Know

- Should all State and Federal Congressional Members be legally protected from the constant pressure their under to accept outside employment, memberships, stock, or direct or indirect campaign donations, subsidies, gifts, or outside benefits during their tenure in office and for five years following their term in office? □ Yes □ No □ Don't Know

Chapter 3
Elections

Questions the Reader Needs to Answer:

- The state should manage the U.S. House and Senate in that they do not report to anyone and that Congress is spending far too much time managing their election or re-election and their salary and benefits programs instead of doing the full-time work they were hired to do? □ Yes □ No □ Don't Know

141

- Should the ugly mud-slinging contests the public experiences in the pre-election debates be brought to an end?
  □ Yes □ No □ Don't Know

- Should state voting programs provide equal and fair campaign financing and supervision for all qualified and approved state and federal candidates? □ Yes □ No □ Don't Know

- Should outside donations be allowed, that subject U.S. political candidates to someone other than the people for whom they have taken an Oath of Office to represent? □ Yes □ No □ Don't Know

- Should the U.S. get all election outside money out of politics since these donations are corrupting far too many unsupervised and federally paid House and Senate members, which destroys the moral and ethical standards of the constitution that should be part of every public official's job? □ Yes □ No □ Don't Know

- Should the people amend the U.S. Constitution to rescind the Electoral College so all citizens can rely on a national popular vote to determine who will become President? □ Yes □ No □ Don't Know

- Should today's corrupted Multi-party election system be allowed to become controlled by corporations, wealthy entrepreneurs, and organizations or other countries? □ Yes □ No □ Don't Know

- Should U.S. citizens amend the constitution to return to a single people party representing "We the People?"
  □ Yes □ No □ Don't Know

- Should the U.S. oversee and coordinate all cost-effective and efficiently run government elections involving all state and national offices while directing all philanthropic donations of money to the state or nation's infrastructure which is currently in a hopeless and neglected state of disarray? □ Yes □ No □ Don't Know

- Should the United States Government's voting system be auditable by using a nationally approved and secure comprehensive computer-based pre-structured touch terminal system that is standard throughout the entire country with a paper-backup and a *"voter's confirmation copy?"* □ Yes □ No □ Don't Know

- Should each election be based on the popular vote and continue to be managed by private citizens that sign today's standard agreement that commits them to remain independent of government or state-appointed officials as well as all outside political factions? □ Yes □ No □ Don't Know

- Should the candidate's credentials include a job application, a comprehensive report on their past educational, mental, physical, family, and social history, and five years of the candidate's tax reports? □ Yes □ No □ Don't Know

- Should the Government of the People require that the President, the Vice-President, the Secretary of State, and all congressional candidates credentials be made available online before the election? □ Yes □ No □ Don't Know

- Should the people require each candidate present and discuss their written statement outlining their primary goals and objectives by both date and cost in a written plan of accomplishment at each debate, stating why they are qualified for the job. □ Yes □ No □ Don't Know

- Should the people require each candidate state how they intend to pay for the cost of their proposals? □ Yes □ No □ Don't Know

Chapter 4
Healthcare

Questions the Reader Needs to Answer:

- Should "We the People" support a single comprehensive

noninsurance healthcare prepayment program under a non-profit private and government tax-supported benefit?
□ Yes □ No □ Don't Know

- Should "We the People" combine the following healthcare facilities, services, and the purchase of products under a single comprehensive, cost-effective nonprofit tax and people supported program?
□ Yes □ No □ Don't Know

Facilities:
All the Armed Services Healthcare facilities
All the Veteran's Administration (VA) healthcare facilities
All the Acute; Obstetrical; Surgical; Pediatric; and Psychiatric facilities
All the nursing and home health care facilities for the disabled and aged.

Services:
The Federal Employees and Politicians Health Benefits insurance program (FEHB)
All V.A. prepayment programs
Medicare and Medicaid
the Affordable Care Act (ACA)
All current state and federal healthcare prepayment services

Products:
Controlling profit-seeking drug manufacturing and healthcare equipment costs through a single universal purchasing system.

- Should citizens that can afford a private paying supplemental profit-seeking health insurance be able to buy additional coverage for elective care treatment? □ Yes □ No □ Don't Know

- Should comprehensive healthcare in the United States be led by professionally trained health care providers that abide by the Hippocratic Oath, not politicians? □ Yes □ No □ Don't Know

- Should the two Multi-party U.S. political systems that have been "Ping – Ponging" health care from nonprofit to profit since 1965, be legally stopped from spiraling health care costs out of control?
  □ Yes □ No □ Don't Know

- Should this nation remain the only nation in the world where profit insurance, the pharmaceutical industry, and a select group of opportunistic Congressmen continue to have no human compassion for the tax-paying sick and disabled when a growing number of financially indigent patients require tax supported coverage for survival? □ Yes □ No □ Don't Know

- Should *"We the People"* support a single confidential patient owned computer-based medical record that uses the professionally designed touch terminal that uses structured entry and bit mapping concepts and *"Code Generation?"*? □ Yes □ No □ Don't Know

- Should *"We the People"* and the U.S. government properly budget for and financially support front-end technical and equipment costs for a single confidential health-record database communications network?
  □ Yes □ No □ Don't Know

- Should *"We the People"* demand top security for a single patient medical record database system? □ Yes □ No □ Don't Know

- Should a computer-based medical record be designed, approved, protected, and maintained by health professionals, before any universal system becomes operational? □ Yes □ No □ Don't Know

- Should citizens be informed that it will take years of cooperative and comprehensive *computer programming* and *operating system design* and *planning* by both the Government and health professionals before a universal medical record computer system can become fully operational? □ Yes □ No □ Don't Know

Chapter 5
Budget and Finance

Questions the Reader Needs to Answer:

- Should the annual budget be monitored and approved by Congress and each department before each fiscal year, and balanced monthly like most successful businesses? ☐ Yes ☐ No ☐ Don't Know

- Should the current disorganized tax system and all budget variances such as congressional favored and unsupervised earmarks require immediate review and revision before being approved?
☐ Yes ☐ No ☐ Don't Know

Chapter 6
Taxation

Note: It wasn't until after the Great Depression and World War II that U.S. taxation began to unravel, as International Corporate bank loans began to open new world markets and exploit cross-border loopholes to avoid trade-tax. The twentieth century's industrial revolution that followed escalated the amount of off-shore wealth to a level that had never involved these new spiraling off-shore "Tax havens." As a result, these tax havens are seriously escalating international corruption as they provide large amounts of international capital to the wealthy CFR members. Conversely, we know from experience that proper and fair taxation is the key to lifting hundreds of millions of people out of poverty, and that tax is the fairest and best sustainable source of finance for any country's development of its people's tax benefits. In fact, the U.S. has already determined that tax-revenues comprise the lifeblood of every country's social contract with its citizens. Therefore, a proper balance needs to be agreed upon (like 80% individual and 11% corporate in the U.S.) and then urgently enforced by all corporations, governments, and societies — and this will be no simple task to accomplish.

An example of a proposed 2018 three level Individual American Citizen Income Tax Rate Schedule might look like this:

146

Tax Rate	Single	Married/Joint & Widow(er)	Married/Separate	Head of Household
I. 0%	$1 to $37,650	$1 to $75.300	$1 to $37,650	$1 to $50,400
II. 25%	$37,650 to $190,150	$75,300 to $231,450	$37,650 to $115,725	$50,400 to $210,800
III. 39.6%	$190,150 and above	$231,450 and above	$115,725 and above	$210,800 and above

I. <u>Pay No Tax</u>:

Pay no tax if a single or married citizen filing separately and earning less than $37,650 annually

If the head of a household earning less than $50,400 annually

If married and filing a joint-return or a widow(er) and earning less than $75,300 annually

II. <u>Pay 25% of Annual Income</u>:

If single and earning less than $190,150 annually

If married and filing separately and earning more than $37,650 but less than $115,725

If the head of a household earning more than $50,400, and less than $210.800 annually

If the taxpayer is married and filing a joint return, or a widow(er) making more than $75,300 but less than 231,450 annually

III. <u>Pay 39.6% of the individual's annual income, or whatever percentage is required that year to balance the budget, including Federal Sales tax, corporate and foreign tax</u>:

Married and earning more than $115.725

Single and earning more than $190,150

Head of a household and earning more than $210.800

If married and filing a joint return or a widow(er) and making more than $231,450

Considering the Congress would approve this type of simplified tax system, you'd need to answer the following questions.

Questions the Reader Needs to Answer:

- Should individual class III taxpayers be required to pay either 39.6% annual tax or the percentage the budget requires each year?
  □ Yes □ No □ Don't Know

- Should the single individual income tax form only list the citizen's total earnings? □ Yes □ No □ Don't Know

- Should Congress eliminate the previous 1040 individual income tax form that has some 79 lines and some 199 related tax forms, comprising some 211 pages of instructions that require tax itemization and the many costly hours of income tax preparation?
  □ Yes □ No □ Don't Know

- Should Corporate annual tax pay a single net profit percentage tax, or whatever percentage is required to meet the budget on every corporate dollar of net profit earned by all profit-seeking Corporations? □ Yes □ No □ Don't Know

- Should the U.S. simplify and implement a single individual and corporate "Tax Standard" that adequately pays the annual budget's total expense promptly? □ Yes □ No □ Don't Know

- Should "We the People" demand a steady, reliable reduction of any further growth in the U.S.'s total debt or % of GDP, which was at $20,538 trillion on the last day of September, 2017?
  □ Yes □ No □ Don't Know

- Should the annual sales tax percent continue on every corporate and citizen's profit-seeking purchase as currently established at the Federal, State, and local level? ☐ Yes ☐ No ☐ Don't Know

Chapter 7
Foreign Trade

Note: The U.S. citizens need to understand that $20 trillion in some 85,000 off-shore Tax-Havens; Shell Companies; Equity Swaps; Avoiding Capital Gains Tax; Evading Estate Tax; Shell Trust Funds; Incorporating; Payments in Kind; Life-Insurance Borrowing; Real Estate Borrowing, are all plaguing every nation. Many systems and individuals also foster this same type of criminal corruption involving the theft of public funds through national and multinational corporations, individuals, lawyers, bankers, and accountants that engage in these illegal acts. Off-shore tax-evasion occurs in the small islands like The Caymans and countries like Switzerland, as well as "International Investment Banks and financial centers" in New York, London, and Singapore and many other areas. All provide and support secrecy and the related perks that only promote more tax-evasion under today's wealth controlled dictatorship style of governance. Tax-evasion is seriously stripping the working class and the U.S. government of their public assets and investment Capital it deprives this once great country of ever reaching a balanced budget without these desperately needed hidden tax-revenues going to the very wealthy one percent, the international corporations, and the U.S. Congress through their many unjust benefits. Fighting this enemy within is one of the toughest "Wars" this democracy has ever faced.

Questions the Reader Needs to Answer:

- Should a new offshore long-term goal for the U.S and the many other deprived countries of the world be promoted to balance foreign trade and replace foreign aid through self-sustaining trade-tax?
  ☐ Yes ☐ No ☐ Don't Know

- Should all democracies be brought together through the UN to cooperate on trade-tax policy, standards, rules, and regulations?
  ☐ Yes ☐ No ☐ Don't Know

- Should the U.S. stop all the current campaign funds and other benefits that the U.S. congressional plutocrats accept to turn their head from their *"Oath of Office?"* □ Yes □ No □ Don't Know

- Should the U.S. promote the UN's *International Law Commission (ILC),"* to bring the following tax avoiding and tax evasion schemes to an end? □ Yes □ No □ Don't Know

  Such as:
  - *Market manipulation and insider buying and selling*
  - *The Fraudulent misappropriation of funds*
  - *Bribing of Congressional members*
  - *Political theft and concealment of public assets off-shore*

- Should the U.S. balance its trade-deficit and tax foreign trade equally? □ Yes □ No □ Don't Know

  Such as:
  - *Lowering the business tax rate from the highest in the world to one of the lowest.*
  - *Eliminating all tax breaks that mainly benefit the special interests.*
  - *Protecting the home ownership and charitable gift tax deductions.*
  - *Repealing the Alternative Minimum Tax (AMT), the death tax, the 3.8% tax that hits small businesses, and investment income.*
  - *Providing tax relief to American families and dependent care, where needed.*
  - *Establish a one-time tax on trillions of dollars held offshore.*

- Should a new single Congress and the UN's ILC promote the following? □ Yes □ No □ Don't Know

  Such as:
  - *Transparency*
  - *International corporate cooperation on tax regulation and accountability*
  - *Open competitive markets based on equitable taxation*
  - *Responsible leadership and enforcement of progressive and equitable tax policy, standards, rules, regulations, and laws.*

- Should the UN's ILC be responsible for taking legal steps to prevent all wars between nations, by enforcing this with a UN multi-nation armed force which all international banks and their CFR owners will legally support financially without profit? □ Yes □ No □ Don't Know

- Should U.S. citizens demand that their sovereignty is restored under a single party electorate so the U.S. citizens of this democracy can once again assume the responsibility for their overall governance?
□ Yes □ No □ Don't Know

Chapter 8
Working Class Benefits

Note: Entitlement benefits include Social Security Benefits; Healthcare and Educational Services that treat all citizens equally; the many facets of this nation's infrastructure such as bridges, post-offices, schools, highways, parks, and the armed services that should be provided equally to all humanity as a non-profit entitlement program. These services, benefits, and even certain products are the earned and tax paid "property" of the working class, the youth and the sick and disabled and the elderly under a Democracy.

Questions the Reader Needs to Answer:

- Should the U.S. Government and *"We the People"* support a qualified state managed SOCC's that protects the entitlement benefits, insurance, and services for the disabled, the elderly, and all of this nation's active workforce benefits, which constitutes the backbone of this nation that lives by equality for all? □ Yes □ No □ Don't Know

- Should the citizen's entitlement benefits and services be subjected to the open market, making an unregulated profit off one's entitlements?
□ Yes □ No □ Don't Know

- Should written constitutional standards and regulations for all entitlement benefits for the people be established under a centralized non-profit structure that is managed efficiently and cost-effectively by

both the State and the Federal Government?
□ Yes □ No □ Don't Know

• Should open competitive bidding be required when the Government is unable to provide the entitlement benefit or service cost effectively?
□ Yes □ No □ Don't Know

• Should the entitlement services and benefits ever be negatively classified as *"Socialized"* or *"Big Government"* programs when these working class benefits are the sole property of every qualified citizen that pays their tax and embraces this outstanding Democracy of "We the People"? □ Yes □ No □ Don't Know

Chapter 9
The Federal Reserve Act

Questions the Reader Needs to Answer:

• Should *"We the People"* repeal the Federal Reserve Act and the IRS code, taking back the ownership of the U.S. Federal Reserve banks?
□ Yes □ No □ Don't Know

• Should "We the People" closely supervises a state-appointed single U.S. Congress with auditable internal controls under a monetary system backed by a value standard such as gold?
□ Yes □ No □ Don't Know

• Should the Public Treasury as outlined in the Constitution once again become responsible for the creation of all money, which must eventually be kept both interest-free and debt-free — thereby establishing a solid pay as you go standard while aggressively repaying the current loans and the nation's out of control and growing deficits?
□ Yes □ No □ Don't Know

• Should the U.S. never again allow private CFR banks or non-government organizations to control this country's money, or ever

again borrow from privately owned profit-centered banks or nations?
□ Yes □ No □ Don't Know

Chapter 10
Debt and Expenditures

Questions the Reader Needs to Answer:

- Should the U.S. Government Accountability Office (GAO) continue to responsibly audit all debt and validate and control all capital and current expenditures while recommending that this nation use only its own money for all expenditures? □ Yes □ No □ Don't Know

- Should the U.S. Government Accountability Office (GAO) continue to plan and manage all capital improvements and infrastructure development responsibly? □ Yes □ No □ Don't Know

- Should Congressional supervision of all debt and expenditures be under a new single party state SOCC system?
□ Yes □ No □ Don't Know

Chapter 11
Contracts

Questions the Reader Needs to Answer:

- Should the U.S. require all Federal and State Contracts universally utilize competitive bidding principles? □ Yes □ No □ Don't Know

- Should all members of the Congress be restricted from either granting or influencing no-bid contracts to their favored corporations which constitutes an illegal conflict of interest?
□ Yes □ No □ Don't Know

- Should all Senators and House Members be restricted from employment for five years after retirement?
  □ Yes □ No □ Don't Know

Chapter 12
Earmarks

Questions the Reader Needs to Answer:

- Should the U.S. legally enforce earmark transparency before authorizing any related legislation and require all public business and policy be open to both public and legal scrutiny under a future State supervised single-party government of the People?
  □ Yes □ No □ Don't Know

Chapter 13
Concerns That Matter

Questions the Reader Needs to Answer:

- Should all U.S. international corporations be educated on the importance and value of not exporting U.S. jobs, thereby protecting this country's sovereignty while discouraging any *"New World Order"* or any *"International Industrial Monopoly?"* □ Yes □ No □ Don't Know

- Should the globalization of the open market encourage worldwide *"Humane Nonprofit Services"* throughout all humankind?
  □ Yes □ No □ Don't Know

- Should the U.S. also protect the Open Market, which involves the selling of competitive and unregulated products in a decentralized open and free competitive market, where the consumer has a choice in what they receive for their dollar — while discouraging international corporate monopolies? □ Yes □ No □ Don't Know

- Should the *"Government Accountability Office (GAO)"* continue to responsibly audit, validate, and control all capital and current expenditures while recommending that this nation use only its own money for such expenditures — while responsibly planning and managing all capital improvements and infrastructure development? □ Yes □ No □ Don't Know

Chapter 14
Personal Issues

Questions the Reader Needs to Answer:

- Should each U.S. state demand their Congressional appointees enforce the many current major personal Federal Acts that have previously been established and enforced, rather than failing to support and uphold these well-defined requirements that were so hard to create after World War II — when Congress still functioned in a bi-partisan manner? □ Yes □ No □ Don't Know

Chapter 15
Policing Other Nations

Questions the Reader Needs to Answer:

- Should the U.S. stop policing or colonizing other countries and significantly reduce all international military bases, while only going to war or fighting terrorism when attacked by another country or terrorist as outlined under UN international law? □ Yes □ No □ Don't Know

Chapter 16
International Law

Note: If this nation is ever to regain the respect it once enjoyed, it needs to identify the criminals that were responsible for the Iraq Religious War. All the related atrocities also need to be sought out and brought to the UN's ILC just as the United States once demanded in the Nuremberg Trials held from 1945 to 1949. The U.S. Protection Act was also intended to intimidate countries that ratified the treaty for the ILC, which currently unjustly proposes that the U.S. Military can rescue any U.S. Personnel brought to trial in the Hague.

Questions the Reader Needs to Answer:

- Should the U.S. abide by the Geneva Convention it previously signed some five times and eventually bring to justice the Iraq war criminals under the UN's ILC? □ Yes □ No □ Don't Know

- Should the U.S. revoke all previous demands for absolute immunity for all U.S. Military personnel and civilian officials, such as the *"Hague Invasion Act"* which President George W. Bush signed into law on August 3, 2002, as the *"American Service-members Protection Act of 2002?* □ Yes □ No □ Don't Know

- Should President Ford's executive order for banning assassinations by any US government formerly known as *"Murder Incorporated"* be re-established and expanded on a worldwide basis? □ Yes □ No □ Don't Know

Screening Presidential Candidates

Balancing what was once known as the "Iron Cross" in the U.S. has long been an important responsibility of every President — requiring they maintain a fair and just balance between the four political powers that represent the four ends of the "Iron Cross." The four ends of the cross represent the *"People,"* the *"Politicians,"* the *"Lobbyists and Bureaucracies,"* and the *"Armed Services."* In 2000, the once "Sacrosanct" Supreme Court was inadvertently added to this balancing act as a temporary fifth appendage when the Court politically, not legally, sent the Republican candidate for President to the White House when the popular vote had elected the Democratic candidate. Previously the President sought to resolve the growing number of two-party liberal and conservative issues that were causing the Senate, the House of Representatives, and the people to become both divided and dysfunctional. Today, it is becoming very apparent that Congress is ignoring the people as they blindly sanction far too many unqualified candidates for the position of President of the United States — one of the most important offices in the world. Both the President and the Congress have failed to properly prepare for this nation's worldwide investment in the globalization of the *"U.S.'s Democracy"* by promoting proper shared principles, policies, standards, and rules of law throughout the world before ever opening the door to the profit-seekers. In other words, the U.S. opened today's large world market — well before the world had prepared for such a huge change. As a result, the entire world is now becoming controlled informally by the wealthy one percent of powerful *"Fascist Leaders"* that are aggressively seeking to gain greater control over the world under a Fascistic, or Socialistic Dictatorship.

In the 2016 Presidential election, Republican candidates employed a non-traditional style of aggressively twittering, mud-slinging, lying, bullying and stirring up fear within a disorganized election. And although these tactics had never before been so overused or even been allowed, these types of psychotic tactics are now terrifying the entire world and urgently need to be evaluated before they destroy this country's once-respected relationship with other nations, as well as humanity as a whole.

Shouldn't it be required that every candidate for this important office be evaluated by an unbiased professional mental and physical screening before ever being permitted even to become a candidate for this most important office? Shouldn't every candidate present five previous years of tax reports and meet a written job description and the signed statement that they will abide by the emoluments clause of their agreement and all qualifications required for all presidential candidates? Shouldn't candidates be required to outline in writing their goals and objectives they seek to accomplish during their time in office, as well as their budget and their projected calendar of accomplishments before ever being allowed to become a valid candidate for President of the United States? Shouldn't we the people of the U.S. have a process that can be rapidly put in place when a President fails to fulfill the demands of the citizens of this country or becomes a *"Demagogic Dictator"* that does not listen to the people but expects the people to listen to him or her? Shouldn't "We the People" demand the President be required to represent the Constitution of the United States by fulfilling the requirements of a Democracy *"Of the People — For the People — under this nation that is governed* by **"We the People?"**

The following serious issue needs open discussion, particularly because the popular vote has failed to appoint a proper President far too often lately and far less than 50% of the population even vote under the current failed system.

Under the current system, a growing number of Americans have all heard enough damning about the U.S., and the resulting loss of our allies already is being felt by the U.S.

It's also becoming obvious the current tactics that seek to destroy our constitutional structure, including the Press; the FBI; the CIA; the private Consumer's Financial Protection Bureau (CFPB); the White House and almost every other highly ethical government department that has been successfully protecting our Democracy for some 243 years. These negative tactics will rapidly destroy any respect the U.S. has justly earned in World

War II and its long history of being the greatest Democracy where the people rule and treat all citizens equally. The citizen's popular vote will also be essential if the U.S. is fortunate enough to turn things around.

Recommended International Policy

- The United States shall assist and support the UN in the very difficult task of developing a Comprehensive Master Plan that is not controlled by the wealthy CFR and attempts to meet the policies and standards that benefit all nations. These policies and standards need to be monitored and financed by each active UN member throughout the world.

- The United States should assist and support the UN's ILC in setting policies and standards for a balanced and competitive industrial economic plan, where every nation can avoid corrupt off-shore tax abuse.

- The United States shall assist and support the UN's ILC in fighting all forms of terrorism, demanding they prosecute terrorists to the fullest extent. The UN needs to assume full authority and responsibility to review, negotiate, and bring to a peaceful resolution all prospective wars before they start.

- The United States should assist and support the UN's ICL in coordinating an international peacekeeping force comprised of a predetermined and equally balanced military force from every participating nation. This international peacekeeping force shall be assigned to maintain *"World Peace"* while methodically investigating and destroying all weapons of mass destruction throughout the world, thereby enforcing the *"Non-proliferation Treaty"* involving Nuclear Weapons.

- The UN should mediate and coordinate a fair and equitable plan for the use of the world's energy resources at the most cost-effective and efficient level for all nations for all nations to participate in equally and follow as each nation seeks to profit equally and fairly in an honest and openly competitive market.

- The UN should resolve the world's dangerous and rapidly growing environmental problems.

- The UN should seek to prevent disease and disability by improving worldwide nonprofit public health.

- The UN should coordinate and enforce standards regarding world trade policy.

- The UN should sanction nations that conduct genocide.

Having Asked for Your Thoughts
I Offer My Opinion

Jonathan Haidt, a social psychologist, in his book, *"The Righteous Mind,"* explains how *"Good people are separated by religion and politics."* What he calls the *"Moral Foundations Theory,"* saying that:

> *"... the vast majority of humans are controlled by our emotions and intuitions. Research indicates that while it may be possible to change our mind based on facts and rational processes, the reality is that we have certain predispositions that guide our everyday actions. Most of our thinking is post facto rationalization. In other words, we do what we do, and then we very cleverly rationalize our behavior."*

It's obvious that in the planned destruction of this great Democracy, we are going to lose everything if "We the People" do not study the facts and then find one's voice and use it!

Living under a system where the *"Winner Takes All"* restricts far too many humans from ever loving their fellow man, and under one's present selfish desire to obtain all those self-serving financial favors humans seem to seek constantly – and which far too often becomes impossible. After all, not having anyone to answer to for one's indiscretions makes one's current life fallaciously easier. But the enemy within is now challenging "We *the People"* to take the necessary steps to protect this great country's Democracy, which involves reclaiming the responsibility and supervision over this nation's political corruption that has invaded the President, Senate, and the House of Representatives. Yes, it's time for this once great democracy to face up to the unbelievable number of out of control and costly benefits the U.S. is losing:

- *The creation of wealth that has become the number one problem in this Democracy's continuance of so many pointless money making wars*
- *The severe and irresponsible congressional overstaffing and lack of supervision*
- *The lack of any understandable or meaningful budgeting or taxation, which is spiraling this nation's deficits out of control*

- *And even more so — the ridiculous wealthy CFR corporate outside factions and international political cyber-attacks in this crazy self-serving "Multi-party" Congressional system that has brought the U.S. to a complete standstill*

During the Great Depression, every citizen of the U.S. came together as one to help solve one of the greatest problems this country had ever experienced. The Japanese sneak attack on Pearl Harbor on December 7th, 1941, which caused every citizen of the U.S. to come together to help solve what was one of the greatest wars ever experienced. "We the People Are Failing" is asking Americans to once again unite as one nation and bond together in one voice to defeat a far greater *"Enemy Within"* that is more dangerous than any other conflict or problem this nation has ever faced. Hopefully, this book will help citizens to see what is going on and help every citizen to become unified and fight as a single nation against this very well organized power that is about to destroy this democracy we all love.

Americans need unity and strength to defeat the current assault on the freedom and equal rights that this nation has successfully protected for some 243 years, during which time we've succeeded in creating the greatest democracy in the world that has until recently protected all the many freedoms we have learned to love. Do not let anyone ever tell you this nation is not great!

However, every citizen is partly to blame since no one can cause the problem all by themselves.

- *Conservatives blame big government and unions.*
- *Liberals blame international corporations and banks.*
- *Voters blame the politicians they appoint but fail to supervise*
- *Politicians take no responsibility for weakening and destroying equality in America.*
- *All of the above factors are abandoning the rest of the world, as this great Democracy once set an example for other nations to follow.*

The U.S. has allowed a well organized *"Fascist"* enemy within, as well as a *"Russian"* communistic country, to control:

- *This nation's elections*
- *This nation's military*
- *Undermine the social media and destroy their unbiased messaging*
- *Divide the U.S. citizens into a conflicting dysfunctional two-party system that must come together as one if the U.S. citizens ever expect to defeat this enemy within*

As a result, the U.S. must reestablish a few of the important things like:

- *A sharp reduction in defense spending and wars*
- *A return to the tax level that previously created a profitable budget*
- *An end to the international corporate offshore tax loopholes*
- *An end to the international religious terrorism killing innocent human beings during the twentieth-century*
- *An end to tax breaks for companies that ship jobs and factories overseas.*

A few things the U.S. must accept and understand are:

- *The U.S. needs a much smaller and less costly single non-partisan state supervised National Congress to efficiently and urgently solve its dysfunctional multi-party problems. Under the current multi-party system, where one party can't win without the other party losing, only leads both parties to adopt policies that split the country.*
- *Healthcare in the United States needs to return to a professionally stable non-profit single healthcare prepayment benefit for all that abide by the Hippocratic Oath.*
- *The U.S. has lost more than 4.5 million manufacturing jobs since NAFTA took effect in 1994, and it's time to realize that most of these manufacturing jobs aren't coming back. Even if companies do shift production back to the U.S., factories are building automated systems that will be employing only a small fraction of the workers they once had.*
- *Under the U.S. current "Multi-party system," one party can't win without the other party losing, and this leads both parties to implement policies that split the nation. The U.S. requires a single party that represents the people, not solely liberal or conservative issues.*

164

- *The U.S. needs to return to a popular vote and replace the current Electoral College that is controlled by a dysfunctional Congress.*
- *The U.S. must stop profitable International Corporations and wealthy individuals from avoiding tax and sheltering income in tax-havens. These tax havens will divert almost $600 billion in U.S. revenue over the next ten years.*
- *"We the People" want Congress to produce an annual balanced budget that pays for universal government benefits that will enhance the citizen's quality of life and the pursuit of happiness.*
- *The U.S. population can demand the U.S. Population vote fairly to Amend the Constitution as outlined as follows in the Declaration of Independence: ...*

> *"Prudence, indeed, will dictate that Governments long established should not be changed for light and transient causes; and accordingly(,) all experience hath shewn (shown) that mankind are (is) more disposed to suffer, while evils are sufferable than to right themselves by abolishing the forms to which they are accustomed. But when a long train of abuses and usurpations, pursuing invariably the same Object evinces a design to reduce them under absolute Despotism, <u>it is their right, it is their duty, to throw off such Government, and to provide new Guards for their future security.</u>"*

The U.S. people have grown increasingly dissatisfied with the performance of the United States Congress, which averaged a pathetic 81 percent in a 2016 pole, and which unknowingly reelects the same members of Congress 90 percent of the time.

Therefore there is an urgency for:

"We the People" to study the facts — find one's voice — and use it to speak out as one!

About the Author

- The **United States Navy Air Corps 1945 -1946**
  I served in World War II and was accepted into the V5 air cadet training program at Pensacola, FL – and went to college under the GI Bill.

- **University of Wisconsin, 1946 - 1950**
  I received an undergraduate degree, majoring in science and physical education while concentrating on pre-med courses.

- **Teacher and Coach - 1950 – 1956 at Canton, high school and then St. Paul Park high school in Minnesota.** Where I taught Biology, Chemistry, Science and Physical Education and coached all sports.

- **University of Minnesota Student -1957-1958**
  I became a student in the number one ranked Hospital Administration Masters Degree Program (MHA) at the University of Minnesota, where I received honorable mention for the James A. Hamilton Award for "Outstanding Student," and became a Fellow of the American College of Healthcare Executives (FACHE).

- **Resident &Assistant Administrator Charles T. Miller Hospital, St. Paul, MN 1957-1964** After completing my MHA Residency at the Charles T. Miller Hospital, (now United Hospitals) in St. Paul, MN - a 440-bed specialist teaching hospital. I was appointed the Assistant Administrator in 1958 under President William N. Wallace, who was also the President and Gold Medal award winner of the American College of Health Care Executives. The Miller Hospital was ranked third in the nation by the Joint Commission on Accreditation of Hospitals (JCAH) back when the JCAH still ranked hospitals.

- **Health Systems Institute, Inc. (HSI) President & Principal Investigator (PI) -1962** to the present.
  In 1961, the President of Miller Hospital asked that I establish HSI, a nonprofit research company devoted to researching the paperless health record involving a nursing/physician pilot research station and numerous corporations, hospitals and medical schools in Canada and the United States while continuing to serve as an administrator of hospitals. I designed nine computer applications that comprise the patient's medical record. I conducted institutes to educate over 5,000 health professionals. I surveyed and consulted with hundreds of hospitals and clinics. I helped Control Data Corporation (CDC) to design and manufacture the first touch sensitive CRT terminal in 1962, the "Digiscribe." The Dgiscrbe was responsible for developing "User Transaction Entry" utilizing "Code Generation," that allowed the user to create their entry transactions for some 90% of the code generated applications HSI developed.

- As **Associate Administrator & CEO at St Lawrence Hospital in Lansing MI 1964-1968 – while continuing as CEO and PI for HSI.**
  Appointed by the Sisters of Mercy Provincialate in Farmington, Michigan as the first lay administrator in their chain of some 350 Mercy Order Hospitals they own and operate – I implemented they're consulting plan to correct their serious financial problem at this 340-bed hospital. I served as a Michigan Hospital Association Board Member and affiliated with the new Medical School at Michigan State, involving a major Nursing/Physician Pilot station that was recognized in May of 1969, by the Department of Health and Welfare (HEW) under contract PH 110-68-47 – Report No. LMSC 682084 National Center for Health Services Research and Development Dept. entitled *"Analysis of Information Needs of Nursing Stations."* This study described the HSI St. Lawrence pilot study as *"a system that will be far-reaching"* and that *"the nurses were pleased with the Digiscribe."* I hired Dr. Eugene Nakfoor, and Dr. John Wiegenstein to provide full-time Emergency coverage at St. Lawrence and was instrumental in persuading them to establish the American College of Emergency Physicians (ACEP). Today, the ACEP saves thousands of lives through a single comprehensive service throughout the U.S. I

also received a Federal Grant to establish the first Regional Mental Health Center in the U.S., which President Nixon later rescinded to save money in 1969.

- **Executive-Vice President of Biomedical Communications Services, Inc. (BCSI) Minneapolis MN. from 1969 -1976** while **Continuing as President and PI for HSI**
  I served as an officer of these corporations and contracted with BCSI to develop detailed application designs for over 50 healthcare applications, including the nine health record applications and its libraries and files. Consulted and advised CDC on their health-related systems, and conducted bi-monthly CDC Seminars in New York City, as well as hundreds of healthcare institutes for BCSI & HSI throughout the United States and Canada. I was ranked the number one speaker in the nation on the paperless health record. Spent a full day discussing the need for a single health care prepayment system with President Ford, and I also met with numerous Senators from 1969 to1976 regarding the HSI systems. I met with Vice President Hubert Humphrey in 1969 to discuss the Navy's request to implement the HSI system. And at the request of Prime Minister *Pierre Trudeau, I* spent a full day with him and more than twenty-five members of his staff to discuss the importance of a single prepayment health care system, which they have now successfully implemented throughout Canada. The Cargill Company in 1976, decided to financially acquire BCSI to stop the HSI regionalization concept of health care in America, so their closely affiliated Pharmaceutical industry would not have to deal with a single prepayment system, and the HSI designs that BCSI acquired from HSI, which were placed in the Cargill vault for safekeeping.

- My numerous consulting appointments have involved very demanding management assignments where I served as Chief Executive Officer, President, and Board Chairman in hospitals and healthcare corporations requiring extensive reorganization — and I also served as a board member for two health insurance companies. I frequently served as an "Expert Witness" involving major health care issues such as serving as a key witness in the infamous Craniosynostosis Surgery law-suit in Colorado that was nationally entitled the "Epidemic that

Wasn't." I've published six non-fiction manuscripts, two fiction novels, and numerous articles on health care — as well as a bi-monthly healthcare newsletter called "Vital Signs." I've served on the NIH committee that defined the Diagnostic Related Groupings (DRG's) and designed and presented the computer-based "Cancer Registry" to the American College of Surgeons. However, HSI still comprises the major part of my career, and from 1984-1989, I attempted to rejuvenate the single healthcare record concept by incorporating **Integrated Transaction System, Inc.**(ITS) in a final effort to try and hopelessly fight the Profit Insurance and Pharmaceutical takeover of healthcare in America.

- **Professional Organizations**: **Active:** Life Diplomat in the American College of Health Care Executives; American Hospital Association; Minnesota Hospital Administration Alumni Association.

- **Previous:**
  Michigan, Minnesota and North Dakota Hospital Associations
  Blue Cross and Blue Shield Board of Directors
  Twin City Hospital Association
  St. Paul, Mn. Chamber of Commerce; Junior Chamber of Commerce; Exchange Club; Rotary
  American Association of Health Education and Recreation Board of Directors in both the Michigan and North Dakota Hospital Associations
  Board Member of two healthcare insurance companies, three hospitals, and three business corporations.

Bibliography

Congressman Louis McFadden, Chairman of the U.S. House Banking Committee and Currency Chairman (1920-31)

Executive Order 10289
Federalist No 10, of "The Federalist Papers," published on November 29, 1787, by James Madison

Federalist Papers: No.9 "The Federalist Papers," The Union as a Safeguard Against Domestic Faction and Insurrection -The Independent Journal. By Hamilton

Forbes billionaires list, the Oxfam report-January 2017.

G. Edward Griffin The Creature From Jekyll Island, published by American Media, 2002,1945,1994)

Joe Scarborough, a former member of the Republican Congress, currently hosting "Morning Joe," on MSNBC

McFadden, Louis T. The Federal Reserve Corporation, remarks in Congress. Boston: Forum Publication Co. 1934)

Milton Friedman's book "Capitalism and Freedom"

President Roosevelt speech at Madison Square Garden in 1936

Senator Bernie Sanders speech at Westminster College on September 21, 2017

The hill.com/blogs/.../politics/267222-the-two-party-system-is-destroying-america jan 28,2016

The State of the Union speech January 31, 2002.: "Bush declares war on the world." www.bushwatch.com/archives-jan06.htm - 225k - Cached

William Ripple, Oregon State University, ecologist

Books by John R. Krismer
Published by CCB Publishing

Our Puppet Government

The New World Oligarchy

The Magic Aquifer

*Conceptual Design Standards for a Single Comprehensive
Health Record Database Communications Network*

We the People Are Failing

Other Books Published

A Prescription for Health Care
— *by Morris Publishing, Kearney, NE*

Should Corporations Practice Medicine
— *by America House Book Publishers, Baltimore, MD*

The Code Generator
— *by America House Book Publishers, Baltimore, MD*

Fair Use Notice

This research manuscript contains copyrighted material the use of which has not always been specifically authorized by the copyright owner. We are making such material available in our efforts to advance understanding of criminal justice, human rights, political, economic, democratic, scientific, and social justice issues, etc. We believe this constitutes a 'fair use' of any such copyrighted material as provided for in section 107 of the US Copyright Law. If you wish to use copyrighted material from this book for purposes of your own that go beyond 'fair use', you must obtain permission from the copyright owner.

www.ingramcontent.com/pod-product-compliance
Lightning Source LLC
Chambersburg PA
CBHW031201270326
41931CB00006B/360